ALLEN
CHIROPRACTIC PC
Functional Neurology

"Brain-Based Solutions with You in Mind!"™

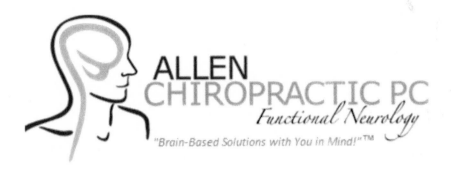

What Your
Brain
Might Say if It Could
Speak

Michael D. Allen, DC, NMD, DIBAK, DABCN, FACFN
Functional Neurologist

What Your Brain Might Say if It Could Speak
By Michael D. Allen, DC, NMD

ISBN: 978-0-9887548-0-5

Second Edition

Printed in the United States of America

If your brain could speak, it might say:

Please be sensible. Do not begin a new health care program or make arbitrary changes to your medications and dosages without first having a conversation with a qualified health professional.

Making "impulsive" decisions to alter your health habits may send chaotic signals that your brain interprets as "repulsive." This may lead to undue stress and complications down the road of life.

Disclaimer

DEDICATION

Throughout my more than three decades of practice as a physician, I realize that none of it would be possible without the guidance of my Lord and Savior, Jesus Christ. I thank Him for His faithfulness each and every day.

And I would be remiss in my thanks if I were to forget the sacrifices my lovely wife Cindy has made to allow me time to write this book. There were many very late nights—more correctly, early mornings—weekends, holidays, and special times that were given up so that I could do this work. Thank you sweetheart!

Finally, but certainly not least, I want to give my special thanks to Kelly Greene, whose know-how helped turn complicated medical ideas into the simplest of phrases, and to Julie Huizenga, a lifelong friend in whom I have the greatest confidence. Thank you both.

What others have said about *What Your Brain Might Say if It Could Speak*:

"The book is written in a style such that you do not have to be a neurologist to follow it or understand it. I have been in the nutrition field for over 40 years and I have never seen such a complete explanation of all the nutrients in one place."

- Sheldon C. Deal, D.C., N.M.D., D.I.B.A.K
Author, *New Life Through Nutrition* and *New Life Through Natural Methods*

"At long last a book that I can recommend our practitioners to read and use as a text integrating nutrition, toxicity, and neurology. In addition it has plenty of hand out advice for patients. I will certainly be recommending it as essential reading to all our natural healthcare practitioners here in the UK and be making it available on our web site at www.epigenetics-international.com.

- Chris Astill-Smith, D.O.
Diplomate, International College of Applied Kinesiology

"Exciting!"

- Christa Hubbard, DC
Functional Neurologist, Fellow of the American College of Functional Neurology (FACFN); Fellow of the American Board of Vestibular Rehabilitation (FABVR)"

"Dr. Michael Allen is a leading expert regarding brain health. His recent book *What Your Brain Might Say if It Could Speak* is a must read for everyone that wants to understand how to improve the health of their brain."

- Datis Kharrazian, DC, DHSc, MS, MNeuroSci
Associate Profession of Neurology, Carrick Institute for Graduate Studies

"As a chiropractor and applied Kinesiologist, the most frustrating part of my practice is the inability to explain to patients the very complex neurological connection with their ill health and spinal subluxations in terms that can be easily understood without needing a major in neurophysiology. Dr. Allen's book provides this as an easy yet concise explanation for both the health professional and the patient. A great read!"

- Eric Pierotti, DC, DIBAK
Immediate Past President, International College of Applied Kinesiology

"Dr. Michael Allen has been a leader in the area of Functional Neurology for over 2 decades. He has always shown an unique ability to take very complex and cutting edge ideas and convey them in an easy and understandable way. Here once again Dr. Allen has done another brilliant job of writing a book that is incredibly interesting, informative, forward thinking, all in an easy to read format. Well done Dr. Allen, this is a must read for anyone with a brain!"

- Robert Melillo, DC, DABCN, FACFN
Affiliate Professor of Rehabilitation Sciences at Nazareth Academic Institute; Senior Research Fellow, The National Institute for Brain and Rehabilitation Sciences; President International Association Of Functional Neurology and Rehabilitation; Co-Editor-In-Chief *Functional Neurology, Rehabilitation and Ergonomics*; Executive Director F. R. Carrick Research Institute; Co-Founder "Brain Balance Achievement Centers"; Author *Disconnected Kids* and *Reconnected Kids*

"In the basic Energy Kinesiology system that is utilized by lay people and practitioners, called Touch for Health, we strive to balance body, mind and spirit. We especially emphasize the muscles and posture, the energy pathways from Chinese Medicine called Meridians, the mental/emotional aspects of our goals, aspirations, and stressful challenges, and our awareness of the food choices we are making, and how they effect our energy and our health. Dr. Allen's new book, *What Your Brain Might Say if It Could Speak*, addresses in depth many of the mechanisms that are involved in each of these important areas. Dr. Allen makes it crystal clear how important it is to feed our brains, and how proper brain balance and function also allows the rest of the body to function as designed. We gain a deeper understanding of the nuances and details of the human 'stress/adaptation' response, and why 'Emotional Stress Release' is so important and profoundly helpful. Our appreciation of the importance of proper brain function is amplified, particularly by the sophisticated and detailed information about nutrition, vitamins, minerals etc., including the important factors that interfere with or enhance brain function, so that the rest of the body can work more efficiently and resiliently. This information, though extensive, is presented in a way that will be beneficial to the lay person as well as the experts in the field, and I believe will be a significant contribution to the understanding, and creation of good health for many individuals, and perhaps many more clients through the improved strategies of their doctors."

Matthew Thie
President, Touch for Health Education, Inc.
Director PR and Research, International Kinesiology College

CONTENTS

MEET
MICHAEL D. ALLEN, DC, NMD

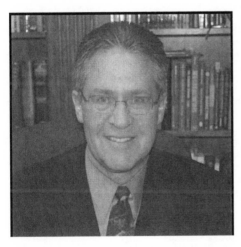

Dr. Michael D. Allen has pioneered several innovative natural healthcare techniques, including how to successfully treat heart and other organ conditions without drugs and surgery. He has unique specialty certification in both functional neurology and applied kinesiology.

Internationally recognized and with over thirty-six years of clinical experience, Dr. Allen has frequently lectured on four different continents and in tens of countries. He specializes in functional neurology, movement disorders, applied kinesiology, and pain management. He has authored several manuals and dozens of professional papers dealing with uniquely human movement patterns and their autonomic concomitants, immune function, learning issues, and several other topics.

Neurology has always been Dr. Allen's forté. He learned clinical neurology from the Carrick Institute for Graduate Studies and became a Diplomate of the American Board of Chiropractic Neurology in 1993. He became a Fellow of the American College of Functional Neurology in 2009.

Dr. Allen's professional education includes graduating with honors from the Los Angeles College of Chiropractic in 1977, and challenging the Arizona Naturopathic Board examination that resulted in licensure as a Naturopathic Medical Doctor (NMD) in 1977. He became a Diplomate of the International Board of Applied Kinesiology (DIBAK) in 1980, of the American Academy of Pain Management (DAAPM) in 1988, and of the American Board of Chiropractic Neurology (DABCN) in 1993. He became a Fellow of the American College of Functional Neurology (FACFN) in 2009. He belongs to the International College of Applied Kinesiology, the Arizona Association of Naturopathic Medicine, and the German Medical Society for Applied Kinesiology (DAGAK, Hon.). He is a past member of the International Chiropractic Knights of the Round Table (1983–2008).

Dr. Allen has served the International College of Applied Kinesiology (ICAK) as the Vice President and Secretary of the American Chapter; and as President, Vice President, and Member-at-Large of the International Council, which oversees eighteen chapters worldwide; he has also served as the Neurology Consultant to the ICAK Board of Examiners.

He is the President of **Allen Chiropractic, PC**—*"Brain-Based Solutions™ with You in Mind"!*™—and founder of HealthBuilderS®, its educational division, in Laguna Hills, California.

PREFACE

The Crimes We Commit Against Our Brains

The "Secret" to Being Healthy

What do you think about this statement: *Our brains are us.*

Does that sound right to you? It rings true to me. Our brains are the tool our nervous system uses to express our needs here on this physical plane.

Every person has a uniquely different genetic background or expression. We all live separate lives, but the fact is that the full complement of our genetic information is greater than 99% similar. Even at the brain's cellular level we are quite similar. In fact, scientists have found that overall we are all about 90% genetically similar, with those 10% differences being quite subtle. Even though we are all so different, we are all very similar at the brain level.

> "No country can be strong whose people are sick and poor."
>
> —Theodore Roosevelt

Have you ever wondered why we humans and other animals have brains? Not all species on this planet have one, so why do we have one? Trees and other plants have no brain. They do not move by themselves. Ask yourself, why do we have a brain? That's too simple. Some might say that we have a brain so that we can perceive the world or to think. I think not. Perhaps the

> Even at the brain's cellular level we are all quite similar.

reason we have a brain is so we can produce flexible and complex movements. Movement is the only way we have of affecting the world around us.

Quieting the Background Noise

Every function of the brain ultimately has to do with the contraction of a muscle. Speech, gestures, writing, sign language are all mediated through the contractions of your muscles. So it is very important to realize that sensory, memory,

> *Motor and sensory feedback signals are not the uncluttered signals you might think them to be. Sensory feedback can be extremely noisy; it can be described as staticky.*

and cognitive processes are only important to drive or suppress future movements. There can be no developmental advantage to laying down memories from childhood if they do not affect the way we move later in life.

Studying vision for vision's sake is not enough. Considering vision as relative to the preprogrammed human movement patterns gives a fresh perspective to what it means to move.

The brain must constantly figure out how to perceive and respond to the world; it has to confront a lot of mechanical and neurological problems. If we reverse engineer any particular movement patterns, we can learn the potential weaknesses of that movement. Movement commands that flow from the brain actually begin as sensory signals sent to the brain from the skin, muscles, and tendons. Closure of this neurological cycle causes muscles to contract and joints to move— and therefore the whole body moves—giving sensory feedback to the brain. The problem is that these motor and sensory feedback signals are not the uncluttered signals you might think them to be. Sensory feedback can be extremely noisy; it is staticky. The "static" inside a nerve is more like the random electrostatic noise corrupting a radio's signal—like tuning an analog radio to a particular station. Moving the tuner slightly toward either side of the true signal leads to greater perception of static, meaning you are not quite focused on the station or target.

> *"Your world is what your senses tell you it is. The limitations of your senses set the boundaries of your conscious existence."*
>
> —From "Sensation and Perception"; Cohen, S, et al; 1984

An often used trick to make this point is to put your finger under a table and try to localize it with a finger from the other hand on top of the table. You might think you have one finger on top of the other, but you will probably be off by several centimeters. You are off the target because of the static in the signals between your sensory and motor systems. This is the same idea as the tests doctors use when they ask you to close your eyes and bring your finger to your nose. Law enforcement does similarly in their field sobriety tests. Further, the outside world contributes its own noise or static by all the changing variables contributed by its changing character. (Our brains have maps that tell us where we are in our environment, but our perception of that environment is only as good as our interpretation of these maps relative to the outside world.) So we move about to the best of our abilities in this whole sensory/movement soup of unlimited ingredients and flavors that we will refer to as noise and static.

The brain puts forth a lot of effort to reduce the level of noise and variability. Insofar as movement is concerned, the brain has an infinite number of choices to perform a particular movement, but many of those choices are dangerous to joint stability. Maybe we do not all move the same way; maybe there is variation in the population. Maybe those who move more appropriately than others have a greater chance for success—athletes are an excellent example. Actually, our movements are extremely stereotypical; we all move relatively the same way. However, our habits dissect our individualities, which lead to our development of self—resolving the conflicts arising from movement's transitional stages—to use a Jungian phrase.

> *There is a direct relationship between the quality of posture and walking patterns, and the ability to think and behave with unique humanity.*

It would be nice if, perhaps through life, movements became better because of various types of learning. While this happens in many cases, in other cases movement is the process that leads to conflict. Neurologically speaking, sensory input to the brain leads to motor output; movement errors are the consequence of sensory conflict. Movement is the result of perception, and vice versa. So what is it about movement that is good or bad? Movement errors become greater as the static increases. Human brains receive sensory input and plan movement responses well before their execution in order to avoid negative consequences. As a result, human brains are there to control movement, and movement influences the brain.

The Most Complex System

The human nervous system is arguably one of the most complex systems in nature. Among all life on the earth, human brains are unique. Humans have relatively large brains that provide for, among other things, rational thought, imagination, free will, speech, and religion. The human brain also affords the ability to write and to achieve an upright posture, the latter being one of the most important human traits.

Our brains control what happens in the rest of our body. There is a direct relationship between the quality of posture and walking patterns, and the ability to think and behave

> *The human brain contains about the same number of neurons as the number of stars in the Milky Way galaxy.*

with unique humanity. The human brain contains over 100 billion specialized cells—called neurons—that control all of our behaviors. Our thoughts, emotions, words, and deeds are all expressions of our brain's function. But it's more than that; human brains are different. Our brains are responsible for coordinating countless processes every second of every day, from muscle contraction to crying.

The whole nervous system contains very important chemical messengers called neurotransmitters, which the brain uses to influence body processes. Neurotransmitters keep your brain's processes intact. They tell your heart to beat, your lungs to breathe, and your stomach to digest. They are also responsible for your opinions, emotions, and other essential functions, including sleep, energy, and fear.

With such a work load, the nervous system must function fluently in order for a person to remain healthy. Unfortunately, stress, poor diet, toxic chemicals, infection, and/or genetics easily disrupt the nervous system. These factors can influence neurotransmitter levels, exposing the brain to either too much or too little, which can lead to feelings of sadness, depression, disturbed sleep, fatigue, behavioral problems, foggy thinking, headaches, or numerous other symptoms.

The good news is that we can resolve these issues. By using a simple exam and making a few changes in strategic areas, functional neurologists can produce profound improvements in a relatively short period.

Unique Humanity

We all have the same basic human neurology. Nerve tracts do not differ from person to person, yet even with our physical similarities and likenesses, our uniqueness comes from our brain. All humans are alike in that we have nerve pathways; however, we each develop our natural abilities in our own unique way. In a sense, we each sculpt our nervous systems by the way we do things and how we live our lives.

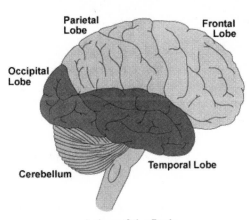

Lobes of the Brain

Brain tissue responds to the stimulation it receives—it is plastic. If a pathway is stimulated, it will respond by carrying a signal. Whether stimulated properly or improperly, the human nervous system will develop relative to the input it receives.

Have you ever wondered what makes one person right-handed and another left handed? Aside from the fact that a right-handed person uses their right hand more, it is the activation of the pathways of right-handedness that encourage these pathways that increase the probability of right-hand use while simultaneously sacrificing the pathways of left-handedness. The converse is true

> *Some of pain's effects on the brain can be reversed if pain is eliminated.*

for a left-handed person. Those pathways that receive more use are encouraged while those that have little or no use waste away; they disappear through lack of use. The way we sculpt, fashion and shape our own nervous systems, and ultimately our brains, makes each of us special. These are the plastic changes that characterize the human brain.

One distinct trait of humanity, the brain's frontal lobe, sets humans apart from animals. In 2001, the journal *Brain* published a study by Dr. Donald Stuss—one of the world's experts on the frontal lobes—in conjunction with The Rotman Research Institute (a part of the Baycrest Centre for Geriatric Care affiliated with the University of Toronto). Dr. Stuss found what could turn out to be the strongest evidence yet that the human frontal lobe differs from those of other primates. The study indicated that the human prefrontal cortex on the right side may constitute the seat of humanity.

The ability to perceive the mental processes of others is considered fundamental to what makes us human and encourages our socialization. This gives rise to our ability to empathize, have sympathy, understand humor, and even perceive sarcasm and deception. These ideas, considered the "theory of mind," are associated with the frontal lobes. Thanks to the research of professionals like Dr. Stuss, scientists are now better able to localize this mentalization ability to the right prefrontal cortex.

In theory all this is good, but what does it mean and how do we use it? Obviously each of us reading these sentences and understanding these concepts has a human brain, but what happens when our brain falters? Is it possible for our brains to get sick? Does it hurt when the brain does not work properly? Can a human brain work in ways other than its original programming? Can it perform in other-than-human ways? These important questions beg for answers, and we will deal with them from a functional neurological perspective as we go along.

Key Lobes

All sensory signals ultimately reach the brain and all motor commands are controlled by the brain. The lobes of the brain make up the brain proper—the cortex. Every facet of life ultimately involves each of the lobes, individually and together at some point. Using the diagram on page 7 ("Lobes of the Brain"), let's

Percentage of total cerebral cortex volume:
• Frontal lobe =   41%
• Temporal lobe = 22%
• Parietal lobe =   19%
• Occipital lobe = 18%

take a moment to familiarize the six lobes and their functions.

The *frontal* lobes are the seat of cognition, reasoning, and memory. The frontal lobes contain the ability to concentrate and attend (i.e., to be present, as to listen, concentrate and focus). They also provide for the elaboration of thought, personality and emotional traits, voluntary motor activity including the motor aspects necessary to generate speech, storage of motor patterns, and voluntary activities.

The most anterior aspect of the frontal lobe is the "human" part. It provides the attention span, perseverance, impulse control, organization, forward thinking, and empathy, and has the ability to feel and express emotions.

A frontal lobe lesion might be detected by the impairment of recent memory, inattentiveness, behavioral disorders, and/or difficulty in learning new information. A person with frontal issues may have a lack of inhibition that displays itself as inappropriate social and/or sexual behavior, and they may have a "flat" affect. A more severe frontal lobe lesion might be characterized by the inability to produce spoken and/or written language. Further, they would probably show a weakness or partial loss of voluntary movement, or a paralysis on one side of their body or in an organ.

The *temporal* lobes interpret and process auditory and visual stimuli, that is, they are generally responsible for receiving and associating sound and vision. As a result, they are involved with long, intermediate and complex memory, and with the retrieval of words that make up language and its meaning. The temporal lobes play a major roll in understanding or taking in what is being said—both with facial expression and decoding vocal intonation—so that our minds can organize sensible utterance. Since the temporal lobes are also involved with conveyed behavior, they play an important role in emotional stability and learning.

A temporal lobe lesion could manifest itself in hearing deficits, agitation, irritability, and even childish behavior. A more complicated temporal lobe lesion may display itself in receptive or sensory aphasia, i.e., the person may be able to speak normally but they are unable to understand language in its written or spoken form.

The *parietal* lobes are connected with the processing of nerve impulses related to the senses—such as touch, pain, taste, pressure, and temperature—and with the comprehensive aspects of language. The complex aspects of spatial orientation and perception also happen in the parietal lobes. The key words for the parietal lobes are processing of sensory input and sensory discrimination.

A person who loses their ability to discriminate between sensory stimuli or who becomes disoriented in their own environmental space could have a lesion in their parietal cortex. They might express their lesion as an inability to read or to locate and recognize parts of their body; i.e., a neglect syndrome. This lesion could even be manifest in the person's inability to recognize self.

The *occipital* lobes are responsible for the interpretation of vision and with the ability to recognize objects. The occipital area includes the primary visual cortex and their associated areas that allow for visual interpretation.

A lesion in the occipital cortex can lead to a loss of vision, or the inability to recognize objects seen in the opposite field of view. A problem here could also be perceived as "flashing lights" or "stars".

The *insular cortex*, (not pictured, but more internal to the temporal lobe) lies between the temporal lobe and the parietal lobe, and handles body representation and subjective emotional experience.

> *The cerebellum contains half of all the neurons in the brain but comprises only 10% of the brain, itself.*

Its functions include perception, motor control, self-awareness, cognitive functioning, and interpersonal experience. It plays a role in diverse functions usually linked to emotion, judging the degree of pain, or the regulation of the body's state of equilibrium.

A lesion in the insular cortex is often difficult to explain because of its detailed neurological and physiological effects involving many and varied aspects of brain function. An insular lesion might be characterized by the loss of balance and vertigo, or as an impaired ability to appreciate the emotional content of music or the functions of language. This issue might be displayed as alterations in the experience of pain, temperature or tactile perception.

The *cerebellum* was originally known as the "little brain." It is one of the most complex parts of the entire human nervous system. It receives input from muscles on the same side of the body, processing it with lightning speed then sending out its influence to the brainstem, midbrain, basal ganglia and various cortical centers to make sure the brain's orders are carried out according to plan.

> *A neuromodulator is a nerve chemical that regulates lots of different neurons. Neuromodulators diffuse through large areas of the nervous system, having an effect on multiple neurons. Examples of neuromodulators include dopamine, serotonin, acetylcholine, histamine, and others.*

The cerebellum is intimately involved with somatic, visual, and other inputs within the cerebellum. Besides synchronizing a multitude of muscle functions, the cerebellum also regulates learning, emotions, and thoughts. As well, it manages the immune system, blood pressure, heart rate, digestion, and many other autonomic functions.

A cerebellar lesion displays itself as a lack of coordination of ongoing movements. The lesion may result in a loss of muscle tone, or disrupt the ability to produce smooth movement on the same side as the problem. These movement errors might include developing a wide and staggering gait, impairment of arm and hand movements, or the inability to stand upright and maintain a direction of gaze. In a very specific type of cerebellar lesion, the eyes may have difficulty maintaining fixation, drifting from a target and then jump back with a corrective saccade, a phenomenon called nystagmus.

Cerebellar patients may have difficulty controlling their gait, or performing rapid alternating movements such as the heel-to-shin and/or finger-to-nose tests. They may have trouble reaching for a target, or display tremors when they move. They may also have impairments in highly skilled sequences of learned movements, such as playing a musical instrument. The common denominator of all of these cerebellar signs, regardless of the site of the lesion, is the inability to perform smooth, directed movements.

Essential Movement

Overall, the human brain loves motion. Movement excites the brain, which sets activity in motion. It makes brains healthier. An active brain is a healthy brain with optimal blood flow and favorable oxygenation—it feels young, acts young, and has a heightened state of focus.

Of that oxygen consumed, 6% will be used by the brain's white matter and 94% by the gray matter.

A healthy brain is better able to experience positive shifts in balance, attitude, attention, memory, organization, self-expression, and vision. If only we could all have healthy brains, but often times we do not. How can we know if our brains are ailing when our brains do not perceive pain? How can we know if parts of our brains are not working properly if we cannot perceive a problem?

When the Insensate Brain Has a Headache

The brain itself is insensitive to pain. One could quite literally poke around in it all day and the host would feel no pain. If it were not for the vast array of blood vessels in the brain, the brain would be pain-

Chronic Pain May Permanently Shrink Your Brain

A recent study (Journal of Neuroscience, Nov. 23, 2006) from Northwestern University indicated an unexpected pain-related brain drain. The study found that brains of chronic backache sufferers were up to 11% smaller than those of non-sufferers. Further, people afflicted with other types of long-term pain and stress might face similar brain shrinkage. In fact, the findings suggested that people with constant pain lose what amounts to an oversized pea's worth of gray matter (the outer layer of the brain that is rich in nerve cells crucial to information and memory processing) for each year of their pain.

The results drew no conclusive cause for the brain shrinkage, but it might involve degradation of neurons, which are the signal transmitters of the mind and body. "It is possible it's just the stress of having to live with the condition," says one of the researchers, Dr. Vania Apkarian. "The neurons become overactive or tired of the activity."

Apkarian also surmised, "Another possibility is that people born with smaller numbers of neurons are predisposed to suffering chronic pain." But some of the differences measured, "must be directly related to the condition."

The research compared the brain scans of twenty-six people who experienced unrelenting back pain for at least a year (and in one case for up to thirty-five years), to those with a pain-free control group. The results showed that pain sufferers had lost 5 to 11% of gray matter over and above what would be expected with "normal aging."

"People who have had pain for longer times have had more brain atrophy," Apkarian said.

The research appeared to make no attempt to correlate brain size to brain function. They did consider, however, that some of the shrinkage might involve tissue other than neurons, and that some of the effects are reversible if the pain is eliminated.

Pain is recognized to be a personal, emotional experience unrelated to the amount of tissue damage. Apkarian points out that, "Different types of pain will have different types of emotional parameters, which will probably result in different types of atrophy—different amounts and in different brain regions."

free. Actually, pain is not perceived as pain until its input reaches the conscious parts of the brain, but those parts have proved themselves formidable in the search for self—a subject for philosophers. Until the conscious brain is reached, pain is more properly classified as nociception (no·ci·cep·tion/ no"sĭ-sep´shun); the relatively slow neural processes of encoding and processing

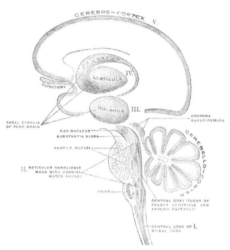

Deep Brain Nuclei and Cerebellum

the stimulation from an actual or potential tissue damaging event.

> *Nociceptive signals are some of the slowest in the whole human nervous system. They travel to the spinal cord and brain at the rate of about 18 inches (0.5 meter) per second.*

Most everyone knows what a headache feels like, so we know that the area inside our head can hurt. I have a lifelong friend whose house backed up to my house. We were brought up together and we are just a couple months apart in age; we went to the same schools together from kindergarten through college. I recall one hot October evening he and I were sitting in my parent's front yard and he asked me, "Michael, what do your headaches feel like?" I was curious because, having been a chiropractic patient all my life, I had never had a headache before. I asked him why the question and he said that his father and mother had headaches as did he and his brothers. He thought everyone had headaches.

Where does this head pain come from? Head pain arises from several places. One theory suggests that it originates from a web-like network of pain fibers that surround the blood vessels of the brain. The tone of the muscles in those vessels is maintained by the autonomic (that part of the central nervous system that controls life-related processes and functions without conscious thought) nervous system, the uppermost representation of which is high in the midbrain; this area receives its main stimulation from muscle and joint signals.

When the muscles in those blood vessels have the right tone, the pain fibers are quiet. As the theory suggests, and as a result of the pressure inside the blood vessels, reduced muscle tone allows the blood vessels to enlarge more than they should. This distends the web-like pain fiber network, firing nociceptive signals down to the cervical

> *The autonomic nervous system is responsible for body processes like blood vessel size, fluid balance, body temperature, sleep and wakefulness, and many others.*

spinal cord and then back up into the brain proper, where the brain's map indicates that something has gone wrong in the specific area of the brain where the vessels are distended. Ouch! That hurts.

> *The respiratory cycles of plants exchange carbon dioxide for oxygen while that of mammals exchanges oxygen for carbon dioxide. These two processes are at the center of life itself.*

Another theory holds that brain pain is triggered by a number of biochemicals that are released at the site of the injury. Some of these biochemicals are histamine, bradykinin, prostaglandin, and substance P, a neurotransmitter or neuromodulator found in the brain and spinal cord. Each of these biochemicals is involved with nociception, stress, and anxiety. Many of these biochemicals are inflammatory—that is, they cause the injury site to swell up. Substance P, for example, also plays a role in influencing the vomiting reflex, defensive behavior, stimulation of salivary secretion, smooth muscle contraction, vasodilation, and changes in cardiovascular tone. Some research indicates it to be increased in the cerebrospinal fluid in those people who have fibromyalgia. Substance P's presence causes sensitive nerve tissue in the affected area to send signals suggesting tissue damage to the central nervous system, which converts them into the experience of pain.

Theoretically, substance P plays a pro-inflammatory role in fibromyalgia. Capsaicin (found in cayenne pepper), on the other hand, is an herb that has

> *Anxiety can contribute to a person's experience of pain.*

been shown to reduce the levels of substance P, probably by causing greater nerve tolerance. Thus, capsaicin is clinically used as an analgesic and anti-inflammatory agent to relieve fibromyalgic pain associated with arthritis, lower back pain, and many types of neuralgia. Clinicians also use it to help ease the pain of migraine headache.

Other examples of herbs that can attack substance P are Ginger, St John's Wort, and menthol from peppermint.

Of all the signals that reach our brain, the majority comes from the muscles and joints that move our skeleton (called *proprioceptors*; pro·pree·o·sep·tors); the most important of those signals come from our centerline spine, and the ribs and muscles that support them, called "a spinal motor unit." Proprioceptor input is the fastest in the whole human nervous system. These signals travel at a rate greater than the length of a football field in one second. If you consider that an average person stands between five and six feet tall, then proprioceptive signals would reach the brain almost instantaneously.

Spinal and rib joint motion, because the central nervous system gives it the highest priority as brain stimulation input, does more for our brains than any other input. By virtue of their neurological input, the ribs, for example, help ventilate the lungs and encourage the healthy exchange of oxygen and other respiratory nutrients to the blood so they can get to the brain. More available air means more potential oxygen to the brain.

When spinal joints and their rib connections move through their full range of motion and according to their original design—that is, when they move

Movement is like food for your brain.

reciprocally—they light up our brains with life-giving oxygen and neurological stimulation. If movement were brain food, then reciprocal joint motion would mean a well-nourished brain. Thus, full motion feeds full humanity.

Muscles Generate Motion

Muscles and bones make up joints, but muscles move the bones, the bones do not move muscles. Receptors (more appropriately, proprioceptors), sensitive nerve endings located inside each muscle and surrounding the joints, detect joint motion. When stimulated, these proprioceptors send their signals to the spinal cord, then on to the different parts of the brain.

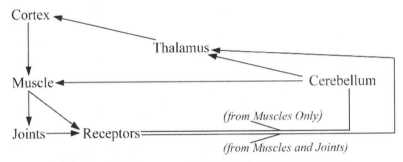

Muscle-Brain Interactions Involves Joints and their Receptors

Because of their unique character, these proprioceptors that reach the spinal cord are able to negate the nociceptive input to the spinal cord before that nociceptive input can be recognized (see the figure entitled, "Schematic of the Spinal Cord and Nerves" on page 272). This healthy neurological competition is a consequence of reciprocal joint motion. Here is the bottom line: healthy joint motion actually knocks out the perception of nociception and/or pain.

Continuing with the above diagram, the muscle aspects of joint motion are ultimately received by the cerebellum, and in response, the cerebellum unconsciously modifies the way these muscles work. These nerve signals travel around and around, up and down the cord, to and from the muscles with continuous stimulation, modification, and activity. At the same time, the cerebellum also sends muscle signals to the basal ganglia and thalamus.

While the cerebellum receives incoming signals from muscle only, muscle *and bone* aspects of joint motion are received by the thalamus (all sensory input must pass through the thalamus except the sense of smell, which goes elsewhere) and, together with the cerebellar signals, the muscle and joint signals finally reach the cortex through the corona radiata—the radiating pathways to brain tissue that look much like the stems of a flower bouquet. The input from the thalamus reaches every lobe of the cortex, connecting each side to the other through the corpus collosum to assure that each of the hard-wired areas might act in concert with the others. From the cortex, the brain's motor outflow controls what the muscles do and how they do it. These outgoing signals go through practically the same coronal channels as the incoming signals do, and they make several homogenizing connections as they pass through the midbrain and brainstem, ultimately reaching the spinal cord.

The moon's gravity is one-sixth that of the earth. Apollo 17 astronauts who spent just over three days on the lunar surface recognized the difference gravity made in their ability to move.

So the muscles receive input from the cerebellum and brain, and these two signals must be reconciled in order for the muscles to work properly. This final reconciliatory phase of muscle function happens in the front part of the spinal cord throughout its course— the final common pathway.

Spinal Joint Lock Down

Healthy spinal muscles (the rotatores, interspinalis, or those deep spinal muscles commonly known as the multifidii; see the diagram on page 19 entitled, *The Deepest Paraspinal Muscles of the Spine*) are termed *antigravity muscles* because they endure the forces of gravity. Their design is a big part of the mechanism that allows us humans to attain and maintain upright posture and bipedal gait. These antigravity muscles—properly called *slow twitch muscles*—are rich in mitochondria and are aerobic, or they require oxygen that allows for their ability to produce ATP (adenosine triphosphate; the body's primary form of energy) over long periods. They are termed "red", or Type II muscles. (See the table entitled, "White vs. Red Fibers," on page 20.)

Instances of locked spinal joints happen all the time—unfortunately, we cannot feel most of them. Spinal muscle spasms can lock the vertebrae into groups of twos and threes within their own normal ranges of motion. These spastic spinal groupings are called *fixations*. Locking the vertebrae together takes away their individual movement patterns and forces them into a grouping that moves contrary to the spine's original design—as one ridged unit rather than allowing each vertebra its own individual range of motion.

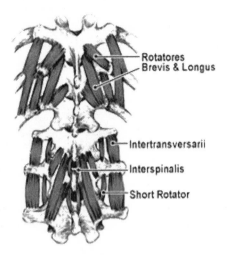

The Deepest Paraspinal Muscles of the Spine

Locked spinal joints quickly lead to both a paucity of mitochondria and therefore the spinal muscle's inability to metabolize oxygen to create energy; the spinal muscles become anaerobic. The spinal muscles begin to look and act more like their white, or Type I, counterparts—also called *fast twitch fibers*—which work with fast bursts of energy and then fatigue quite easily. When the spinal muscles fatigue they fail, and their failure results in vertebral lock down. The brain pays the price for vertebral lock down because the individual signals that would have otherwise been sent to the brain remain silent. That joint silence is detrimental to healthy, or preprogrammed human brain function.

> *Muscles use calcium to contract and ATP energy from mitochondria to relax. Spasmed muscles are actually mitochondria-poor and energy-starved.*

Furthermore, when spinal joints become stuck, the spasmed muscles cannot perform useful work. The muscles are said to be working insofar as they are in spasm, but spasmed muscles are ineffective both relating to their movement and their sensory input, and that vicious cycle perpetuates their spasm.

There are two reasons for muscle atrophy: disuse and denervation (e.g., an absence of nerve signal to and/or from a muscle itself). Disuse atrophy will return with proper stimulation and rehabilita-

Chiropractors used to speak of pinched nerves, but nerves rarely get pinched. Medicine stayed away from the term because they thought it was archaic. More recently, medicine delights in the term while functional neurologists have moved on to more neurologically explicit terms.

tion, but denervation persists. Denervation atrophy is related to actual nerve pinching or other types of real nerve trauma. While both types of atrophy should be treated by a doctor right away, in the absence of denervation atrophy, most any perceived pinching of a joint (usually of a spinal joint) means that there is inappropriate joint stability—a reduction of joint steadiness secondary to disuse atrophy—that allows the nociception to reach conscious levels and be perceived as pinching.

Do not allow your spinal joints to remain in lock down! It only takes six to ten days for an inactive muscle to lose half its ability to do its job of moving bones. In the *next* six to ten days they lose half of their remaining ability. Statistically, after a month, a muscle can lose up to 90% of its functional ability, and then the joints get sloppy. What a crime!

Move It or Lose It

White vs. Red Fibers

White	Red
Type I muscle	Type II muscle
Fast twitch or contraction	Slow twitch or contraction
Anaerobic	Aerobic
Few mitochondria	Copious mitochondria

When the vertebrae get locked down, the individual segments get stuck within their normal range of motion, and only that input from the moving parts above and below the fixation reaches the brain. Movement that never happens sends no signal—the brain forgets about it, and misses out on the stimulation it would have otherwise had. This is where the saying, "Move it or lose it!" fits nicely.

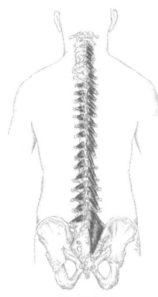

**The Spinal
Stabilizing Muscles**

Since the intent of the spine is compromised by spinal fixations, the joints above and below the fixation must take up the slack, and this contributes to their structural breakdown. These joints not only have to manage the stress of their own movement, but they must also take on the added stress of the fixated joints. This results in spinal pain, spinal muscle strains, ligament sprains, and degenerative joint disease characterized by arthritis.

Remember, when we say that a spinal joint is stuck or "locked down" within its normal range of motion, we mean that it can move one way but not another. Compounding its crime, the brain signal that would have come from the lock down remains silent through the range of motion that is locked, robbing the brain of its rightful input, perpetuating the abnormal motor output to the spinal muscles. Furthermore, the area in line for the secondary benefit of the missing signal also suffers. Guilty as *un*charged.

How Joints Become Stuck

If your brain could speak it might ask, "Am I the guilty culprit?"

The human nervous system—the brain and spinal cord being the central nervous system, and the rest of the nerves making up the peripheral nervous system—is designed to work in a specific, pre-programmed way. Although we as humans are the sculptors of our own nervous systems in that we define our distinguishing natural abilities, the human brain and the nervous system are hard-wired to operate in a uniquely human manner—its display is predictable, and any unanticipated display is pathology.

Sadly, this silent thief—pathology—operates so cleverly that we are oftentimes unaware that our bodies are under attack. Thus, we may be unwitting accomplices to the crimes being committed against our own brains.

Gravity Made Me Do It

Working at a computer station that demands constant turning in one way or walking with one leg that is even slightly shorter than the other are just two examples of activities that can produce more muscle tone—or more pull—on one side of the body. Over time, the sensory signals related to asymmetries of this sort result in irregular—or unpredicted display—in the brain. As gravity is the only constant on this earth, any activity that favors one side of the body over the other can eventually lead to structural imbalances.

There are many other common situations in our daily lives that lead to brain asymmetries. Remember, the more brain input received from one side of the body has a very high probability of causing tighter muscles on that side of the spine, and this results in vertebral lock down within their normal range of motion.

The Quiet Thief

Some areas of the brain require excitement, and others need it quieter. There are also times when certain other areas of the brain need to be "excited" so they can then "quiet" other areas.

It is a fact that vertebrae stuck in lock down steal input from their rightful manager—the brain. An unnaturally stimulated brain reacts in peculiar ways. So, what happens if one area of the brain that needs to be excited in order to quiet another area of the brain is robbed of its signal and remains unstimulated? Remember, any unanticipated display is pathology, so the second area would remain inappropriately excited—leading to neurological activity that otherwise would

> *What good is it to know the anatomy of the multifidii (spinal muscles) without clearly understanding what to do with them when they are dysfunctional?*

not have happened. Get the picture? Guilty as *un*charged on a second count!

Hunger Strike

A healthy, well-fed brain is a neurologically typical brain. It has optimal signal input and is stimulated according to its preprogrammed symmetry. In general, a "neuro-typical" brain controls the activities beneath it. Let me say that another way. The brain's output keeps the successively subordinate areas focused on managing the proper signals at the proper time.

Likewise, the starved brain—one on a signal-poor diet—abandons interest in the other parts of the body. An unhealthy brain simply does not have enough appropriate nerve signal to keep the brain regimented with sufficient ability to influence normal bodily processes. The person with the starving brain may not even be aware that their brain is in distress because they have lost their ability to realize; however their body displays the nervous system's internal struggles through muscle dysfunction. Static jams the human nervous system's channels! The signals go haywire! There are no appropriate controls! A starving brain cannot perceive what it cannot receive.

Remember, spinal joints that are stuck in lock down create flawed brain function. A signal-starved brain is subject to signal imbalances—muscles turn on when they should be off, and remain off when they should turn on. Joints pull when they should relax, and relax when they should pull. This can lead to structural imbalances and increase the potential for injury. We see this all too often in our offices.

Let's Take a Walk

Another trait of our unique humanity is our bipedal posture—standing upright on two feet. It is our spinal muscles that enable us to stand up straight. They are designed to resist the effects of gravity all day long to maintain an upright posture. These "antigravity" muscles are under involuntary control of the cerebellum, and are located for the most part on each side of the spine and hips. They help us to walk, maintain posture, and perform coordinated movements.

The spinal muscles must be aerobic—that is, they *require* the presence of oxygen—to endure the effects of gravity throughout our waking hours. Antigravity muscles are the same as the muscles that surround the spine. They have the richest concentrations of mitochondria—the cell's powerhouses—to produce the necessary energy for their staying power.

How Gravity Wins

As we learned earlier, when one-sided movements (such as repetitive desk work) generate imbalanced signals that reach the brain, the result is a tightening up of the paraspinal muscles. At this point, the signal degrades, the muscles quiet, the brain loses contact with the input from the paraspinal muscles, and the spinal system—and therefore the rest of the structure—fatigues.

Furthermore, the mitochondrial populations in the antigravity muscles fail and they lose the ability to generate the energy they need. Sadly, muscles designed for endurance begin to resemble

The original concepts of functional neurology were developed by my good friend and teacher, Professor Frederick Carrick, of the Carrick Institute for Graduate Studies in Cape Canaveral, Florida. Prof. Carrick's original ideas have progressed relative to his vast clinical experience, innovative research, and continuing deeper understanding of the human nervous system's function.

Functional neurology is the multidisciplinary study of the inter-relationships of an individual's nervous system within the context of their greater health. It considers that a person's functional state is generally determined by the quality of their brain's input and the clarity of its output as well as the supply of nutrients and oxygen that reach that person's nervous system.

Functional Neurologists consider that the functional state of a person's nervous system will impact all related systems that are anatomically or embryologically related. They use these relationships to effect a positive neurological change using intrinsically and/or extrinsically generated stimuli that build functional neuroplasticity within the dysfunctioning nervous system, thus improving the neuronal performance of the individual as a whole.

muscles that do short—anaerobic—bursts of work (a metabolic process that happens *without* oxygen). They lose the ability to resist gravity, they fail more easily, and the proper upright posture is more difficult to maintain.

So we can see that a compromised structure fails easier, joint function is impaired, and the brain receives inconsistent and asymmetrical signals. A brain in chaos lacks its underlying humanity. Coordination suffers, and this threatens our balance and bipedal stance, increasing the potential for injury.

Did you know that the highest occurrence of accidental death comes from incidental falls? It is absolutely true! The spinal column is made up of twenty-four moveable bones connected by twenty-seven longer muscles and various smaller and deeper muscles on each side—the paraspinal muscles—that run the whole length of the spine. They relay information about body position and balance directly to the brain. Any spinal movement error causes the wrong message to reach the brain, resulting in symptoms of imbalance, and any paraspinal muscle imbalance can lead to a spinal movement error. These movement errors are called subluxations, displacements, or misalignments of the spine. A functional neurologist recognizes how to deal with these subluxations to restore spinal balance and heal the brain.

Moreover, certain areas of your brain control how your spine moves. Any dysfunction in these areas will display itself in spinal distress. Since the spine and brain are so closely linked, any spinal trouble will manifest itself as brain trouble. These and many other issues like them are the specialty of functional neurology.

Despite occasional back pains or headaches, the majority of spinal subluxations are painless. But when we do realize the pain, all too often it is the result of unresolved spinal movement errors and chronic joint breakdown. The ensuing proprioceptive chaos allows the nociceptive signals to make their way through the spinal cord and ultimately reach conscious cortical levels where we realize pain. Many pain sufferers wait to see if it will go away by itself, and if it does, they think they have been healed. But be careful, the healing has oftentimes not occurred.

When spinal joints become stuck, atrophy quickly takes its toll on the paraspinal muscles. At this point, the entire centerline structure breaks down vertebra-by-vertebra and group-by-group. One fundamental rule in functional neurology is that centerline structures relate to centerline organs, and centerline organs relate to centerline structures. So, if the spinal motion segments are allowed to break down, then so does your brain, your posture, your gait, and your consumption of oxygen. Because the spine and all the spinal joints run along the centerline of the human frame, once the spinal joints break down, nothing else can provide structural stability.

Finally, the ribs attach to the thoracic vertebrae—those vertebrae from your shoulders to your lower middle back. Their attachments are meager but they are nonetheless functionally important. Rib motion contributes to the breathing mechanism, and when they get stuck it reduces the potential for oxygen to reach the brain, starving the brain of one of its key nutrients. If the movements of the spine and rib joints are considered brain food, then allowing spinal and rib joints to remain stuck means we are starving our brains.

Fixing Stuck Joints

There are ways out of this brain-spine mess. Typically, people turn to massage and physical therapy to loosen their stuck joints. They figure that it makes sense to get their muscles relaxed and their joints moving again. But if these people first turn to physical therapy, perhaps they do not fully understand what functional neurology can do for them.

> *Restricted spinal joint motion leads to brain starvation.*

Despite the fact that the skin is made up of exactly the same components as the nervous system, i.e., surface ectoderm, physical medicine—physical and massage therapies, yoga, Pilates, rolfing, etc.—cannot appropriately stimulate the higher brain levels necessary to achieve all the desired cortical results because they can-

> *If a door hinge gets a catch, the door cannot swing as freely as it should. The same is true of the spinal column. If a vertebra gets stuck, it cannot move as it should, and this can have brain-centered consequences.*

not affect the deepest spinal muscles. Physical medicine is unable to deliver the appropriate fast stretch to the deep spinal muscles—the paraspinal muscles that connect vertebra to vertebra. Only properly trained and licensed Functional Neurologists are taught the dynamics of proper and coupled fast-stretch structural adjustments. However, once the proper adjustment has been made then physical medicine techniques may be appropriate, under specific direction of the doctor, to keep the bones in place by rehabilitating the joint motion and increasing stability.

Like the hinges on a door, spinal joints need their own free range of motion. Exercise alone cannot relieve stuck spinal joints because spinal joints are not under voluntary control. No one can voluntarily move or relax one vertebra relative to

> *A plastic brain is changeable. That truth is being used to develop a novel generation of educational and rehabilitative methods for enhancing human mental function, both in children with learning disabilities and aging adults.*

another; it is neurologically impossible. Humans are not wired that way. In fact, exercising improperly can *create* spinal joint problems because improper training results in inappropriate plasticity.

Correctly releasing stuck spinal joints with a fast-stretch manipulation requires specialized coupled chiropractic techniques. When executed properly, coupled spinal adjustments can re-ignite the brain, releasing the muscles they control, and restoring the human nervous system to its original design.

After the right adjustment, specific nutrients can reinforce the proper muscle function and spinal stability that help the adjustment hold. Rehabilitation exercises—such as crawling (yes, crawling), walking, reaching, tumbling, as well as resistance exercises, all build a stronger, healthier spine, which quickens the brain. At **Allen Chiropractic, PC**, we specialize in a wide range of techniques from traditional chiropractic and functional neurology, to several innovative techniques that are on the leading edge of alternative healthcare.

Our brains want to grow and learn; they are plastic. A plastic brain responds fluently. It is moldable, readily sculpted relative to the signals it receives. A plastic brain expresses itself beautifully. It will respond to its environment in either a human way or in a dysfunctional way. The human way is the healthy way; the dysfunctional way is full of pathology. Which do you choose?

Building spinal joint stability encourages our human nature, allowing our brains to work according to their original design. A healthier brain means improved blood flow, increased oxygenation, heightened focus, and an altogether higher quality of life—an optimally human life. *Got motion? There's a brain to build!*

OVERVIEW

"What Your Brain Might Say if It Could Speak"

Developing good health is not just about nutrition. Good health is not just a quick pill for every ill. The "pill for every ill" mindset that believes pills make everything better can eventually lead to trouble further down the road of life.

Good health does not just happen; neither does proper nutrition. Both require awareness and determination. Eating right and taking supplements are good practices, but something else needs just as much attention—our neurological health. Nerves are often taken for granted because few people are aware of what they really do. Remember, the nervous system controls all body functions, and this also includes influencing how body tissues use the nutrients they receive. And when it comes to brain health, neurology is king!

Who Else Wants a Healthier Brain?

The sensation of motion is like the other five senses. Okay, well perhaps motion or movement is more a *result* of the other senses acting in unison than it is a sense of its own. Nonetheless, movement brings sensation to the cortex. People often do not give much thought to their ability to move

Nutrition, unlike what most doctors think, is not the key to treating patient problems but it is essential for the rehabilitation of their issues. Most people's problems are physiological rather than nutritional.

29

until that motion breaks down or their bones become too thin to bear their weight. Muscle soreness, general fatigue, and various aches and pains can keep one sidelined, sometimes for days at a time.

A long while back, a radio talk show host presented me with a challenge. He caused me to ponder what my brain might say if it could speak. While he continued his discussion, I sat there remembering all sorts of things I have "heard" patient's brains say. I came up with so many answers that I hardly knew where to start.

Oh, the ideas that went through my head. There were so many! When it came right down to it, I had four answers: *"I can't breathe!"*; *"I can't take it anymore!"*; *"I lost the words!"*; and *"Stop the static!"*

The primary goal of the brain is survival. It must endure at all costs. Neurological survival requires three things: available oxygen, plenty of fuel in the form of glucose delivered to the tissues by the blood, and a specific type of stimulation that enables all of its requirements to function properly and ensure healthy survival. When all its needs are met, the brain is happy; however, the lack of any one (or any combination) of these three things means that your brain will not function according to its original design, which may cause it to age too quickly.

"I Can't Breathe!"

The brain contains the most oxygen-sensitive tissues in the whole body. Without access to available oxygen, brain tissues deteriorate quickly. It must be able to breathe. But how can we say the brain "breathes" if it does not have lungs? We will discuss the importance of getting blood to the brain and how that helps the brain to breathe.

Among the tissues of the brain, those of the cerebellum and basal ganglia are the most sensitive to oxygen levels. They and the brain proper need oxygen to meet the metabolic demands of processing the

The human brain requires oxygen from the blood in order for the brain to perform according to its original design. The brain is unable to switch from aerobic metabolism to anaerobic metabolism because the brain has no means to store long term energy.

amount of information received. The cerebellum interprets input solely from muscles and then sends its analyses to the thalamus. The basal ganglia also feeds information to the thalamus. The thalamus receives input from everywhere—muscles, ligaments, joints, skin, etc. All incoming signals that ultimately reach the brain (except the sense of smell) blend within the thalamus and then are sent to the cortex in order to generate a motor response. The input from the cerebellum, basal ganglia, and thalamus must work together. Without oxygen, their functions break down quickly. These three areas can tolerate low normal blood oxygen levels with subtle changes, but if the blood oxygen level drops too low over too long a period of time, then their tissues will degenerate—hastening the aging process, structural breakdown, and senility—and if oxygen levels drop below critical levels for just a few short minutes, the result may be brain damage or even death.

> *For centuries, scientists have said "the dose makes the poison," meaning too much of any chemical can be toxic. Likewise with oxygen: too little or too much can "poison" the brain. The hand of time delivers the deadly dose.*

There is no doubt that a breathing brain needs the proper nutrition. It also needs neurological input to help its sensitive receptors read the blood's oxygen and carbon dioxide levels in strategic areas. For example, if the signals to one such receptor found in the neck become chaotic, the signals might provide the brain with faulty information, causing the brain, in turn, to make blood vessels too big or too small. Blood vessel size affects blood pressure, adapting blood flow to the brain.

"I Can't Take it Anymore!"

> *One basic chiropractic tenet is, "too much or not enough nerve energy is disease." Remember, moderation in all things is wise. Even drinking too much water can be deadly.*

When the brain says that it can't take it anymore, it is speaking of the toxic insult of poor nutrition and the incomplete elimination of wastes, which compromise tissue quality and clog neurological communication channels. Toxins build up for many reasons, but mostly because of dietary or metabolic error—or from unnecessary drugs and medications.

> *The right amount(s) of essential nutrients plus a high rate of metabolic activity equals a highly efficient brain.*

Balanced tissues use nutrients as they should, and unbalanced tissues use them incorrectly. While the first case might represent the smooth flow of metabolic consumption from one point to another, the second might represent the accelerated use, or conversely, the backing up of those same metabolic pathways, leading to toxic buildup.

Imagine that the metabolic channels are like rivers flowing throughout the body. Just as water in a river flows from one place to the next, metabolic byproducts flow from one molecule into another with the help of vitamins, minerals, enzymes, and other cofactors necessary to transform the metabolites until they reach their end and are finally eliminated from the body. And just like a river, these metabolic flows can become dammed up by the absence of their essential components or the presence of toxins, creating a pooling upstream and a trickling downstream. This is another way that toxicity increases within the body. When the metabolic channels become clogged there can be too much of

Metabolism of L-Tryptophan into Serotonin

one substance and not enough of another, making the tissues tired and tainted.

There are many examples of how a metabolite changes from one molecule into another. (Do not get lost in the biochemistry figures on page 32. Rather, observe that one product transforms into another.) Under certain metabolic conditions, the amino acid L-tryptophan gets metabolized one way to become niacin. Via other metabolic pathways, that same tryptophan molecule converts into serotonin and then into melatonin. These transitions depend upon the intervening factors, the metabolic needs, and the presence (or absence) of essential nutrients to drive the metabolism in one way as opposed to another. The conditions that cause the metabolic flow to go in a specific direction depends upon many different factors.

> *Lingering toxins forge their own metabolic paths, leading to potentially deadly complications down the road.*

Another example of these metabolic changes is "trans" (bad) fats that can alter the way nerves work. They change a nerve (or any) cell's structure, which alters both the nerve's ability to transmit a nerve signal and can impede the way nutrients enter or wastes leave the cell. Therefore, trans-fats hinder cellular performance, and those cells can suffer for a long time, and even die.

An article from the *American Journal of Clinical Nutrition*, (entitled, "Can nutrient supplements modify brain function?") found that diet influences the chemistry and function of both developing and mature brains. As a result, investigators, physicians, and regulatory bodies have supported and encouraged the proper use of nutrition in the treatment of disease.

> *"Manufractured": a major trend taking place today in visual and material culture; the radical appropriation of consumer goods as raw material for art- and object-making.*

People often begin taking nutritional supplements by their own accord when they or someone they know took the nutrient for a similar condition and had positive results. Typically, if a nutrient works well for a specific condition, people tend to take more of it in the hope of achieving better results. However, if a little bit is good, then a lot is not necessarily better. A stronger dose does not necessarily lead to a better outcome, in fact, it can even be dangerous.

While recently lecturing in Moscow, Russia, one doctor was surprised to hear me say that eliminating "static" in the human nervous system reduced or eliminated the need for so many supplemental nutrients.

He said he used the techniques I taught him on four Olympic athletes and they worked quite well, but the athletes did not seem to need as many supplements as they did before. He asked if I see this in my practice. I replied, yes, this is common. Once the brain is in sync with its original design, the biochemical aspects of brain function take on a whole new and appropriate character.

This illustrates how an imbalanced nervous system either accelerates or slows the consumption of particular nutrients. Resetting the nervous system according to its original schematic may eliminate or reduce the need for so much supplementation. Balancing the nervous system can simultaneously balance the nutrient delivery systems and restore optimal performance.

The marketplace eventually encourages companies to manufacture supplements that are broken down to their purified state—this might be better known as "*manufracturing.*" This is what synthetic vitamins are all about. The nutrient's active ingredients are separated out—distilled or fractionated—from the original complex, and the rest of the molecule is discarded. Sadly, there can be many heretofore unknown nutritional factors that are cast off as waste. In many cases, these same unknown factors are the same ingredients that are necessary to modify the effects of the purified product. What used to be a whole nutrient with all the essential components for its breadth and depth has now become a refined substance—vitamin, mineral, cofactor, etc.—with an increase in potency that nature never intended, and that the body is ill equipped to handle. This can lead to unanticipated adverse effects much like a pharmaceutical. The B-vitamins are an excellent example. As we shall see, there are many B-vitamin factors, but since many of them are unrecognized as useful to humans, they are discarded by vitamin companies and regulatory agencies as unnecessary.

In the short run, people believe they are helping themselves, but how can they truly know what their bodies need if their own pathology is interfering with their ability to accurately perceive how they feel? They actually have no way of knowing what they are doing unless they have overt symptoms. Actually, most people are unaware that many of their supposed symptoms are the side effects of their naked nutrients. They seek professional care for what could be managed by simply discontinuing the fractionated supplements and *resupplying* their body with

> The catecholamines are the "fight-or-flight" hormones released by the adrenal glands in response to stress; the most abundant catecholamines—epinephrine (adrenaline), norepinephrine (noradrenaline), and dopamine— all come from the amino acids phenylalanine and tyrosine. The opioid peptides (which mimic the effect of opiates in the brain) may be produced by the body itself, like endorphins, or be absorbed from partially digested food. Brain opioid peptide systems are known to play important roles in motivation, emotion, attachment behavior, the response to stress and pain, and the control of food intake.

the essential nutrients that have been taken away.

> A typical protein is a complex macromolecule made up of unbranched chains of 200-300 amino acids that include carbon, nitrogen, oxygen, hydrogen and sulfur. Protein is a fundamental component of all living cells. Proteins are required to produce, maintain and repair bones, hair, skin, muscles and other organs. Proteins play a significant role in the production of hormones, enzymes and even genes. Proteins can be obtained from various foods including dairy products, eggs, meats, fish, vegetables and legumes.

The brain needs a clean work environment. It has a very high metabolic rate and consumes more glucose and oxygen than any other organ. Since all metabolic processes generate wastes, the brain— because of its high metabolic rate—is especially susceptible to toxicity if the wastes are not removed quickly. The brain's environment must be squeaky-clean for it to work at its highest level.

If toxins linger in the brain too long, they create their own problems. Retained wastes and toxins clog up the system, generating more wastes and toxins, and inefficient purging hampers toxin breakdown. The same results follow when the nutrients that would otherwise control a metabolic path are removed or missing from foods, or when a vitamin's potency increases because of its purification by distillation or fractionation.

The liver stores many nutrients, and it is the major organ of detoxification. It processes metabolic wastes and pollutants from the blood that come to it from all over the body. Generally, the liver has two detoxification phases. Phase one breaks toxins apart, and phase two combines the end products of the first phase preparing them for elimination. If the first phase of detoxification succeeds but the second phase fails, the toxins from the first phase can get back into the system where they often have effects more toxic than the original products. So it makes sense to be sure your detoxification pathways carry through to completion.

> Neurochemicals are uniquely designed to relay, amplify and modify the nerve signals that occur between one neuron and another.

An unhealthy diet—one poor in fiber, deficient in minerals, and rich in simple sugars or refined carbohydrates, additives, colors, preservatives, etc.—tends to cause liver congestion. A stagnant and congested liver can cause symptoms like skin problems, poor eyesight, hair loss, hemorrhoids, and much more.

Besides the liver, the kidneys and skin also eliminate toxins from the blood. In fact, the skin, which is the largest eliminative organ of the entire body, shares its same basic tissue as the nervous system— called surface ectoderm. The health of the skin can hint at the health of the nervous system. Touching the skin stimulates immediate and profound nervous system changes; keeping the skin clean also helps keep the nervous system clean.

"I Lost the Words!"

The brain speaks in *"neurologese"*—a brain-specific language that blends neurotransmitters and neurochemicals into "words." The brain's internal conversation requires the right timing if words from one part of the brain are to be "heard" in another. The words and the timing of their delivery keep the brain from becoming confused. If the brain's words become confused, then the brain loses track of what it is saying and how it says it. A good analogy might be that your brain's natural dialect of neurologese changes to something alien.

While neurotransmitters originate from within the nerve cell itself, neurochemicals exist outside the cell, relaying, amplifying, and modifying signals between one neuron and another, or between one axon and another. Neurochemicals, including neurotransmitters (and other neuroactive molecules, like catecholamines and opioid peptides), constitute the *language of the brain*.

Getting a neurotransmitter or a neurochemical from one nerve cell to another is like watching a horse race. When that starting bell rings, the horses run with all their might, each one trying to cross the finish line first. In much the same way, when a group of neurotransmitters are stimulated, they each strive to reach the next nerve first, making that subsequent nerve send its signal. When the right concentration of neurotransmitter substance reaches the next nerve, then the designed signal continuity is maintained; however, a short supply of that neurotransmitter can cause the nerve to remain unstimulated. That can cause confusion because a nerve that was originally intended to be stimulated, remains silent.

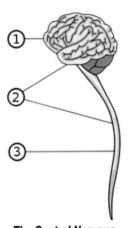

The Central Nervous System:
1. Brain; 2. Central nervous system: brain and spinal cord;
3. Spinal cord

While we know that certain drugs can change the way the brain works, they actually work by changing the concentration of neurotransmitters in the tissues. Scientists are finding that science can also influence brain function by managing the way the brain makes proteins from amino acids. A brain's diminished ability to build proteins affects its response to neuroactive drugs, while increasing protein synthesis increases its response to the drugs.

> *The difference of one amino acid in a protein sequence changes the way that protein works.*

When the brain has a neurochemical imbalance (i.e., trouble with its "words"), the result is chaotic chatter. Balancing neurochemicals—normalizing their production and controlling their longevity—depends upon a fluent nerve signal. As nerve signals change, so do the ways the neurochemicals are generated, which can change the way the person's nervous system works. The amount of physical stimulation and the quality—and quantity—of nourishment both influence neurotransmitters, leading to functional brain changes.

"Stop the Static!"

The first three "Brain-Speak" topics deal with the brain's metabolic issues and nutritional needs. They discuss how the brain needs oxygen, the importance of detoxification, and the

> *Your brain must be aerobic to perform optimally. Anything less is pathology.*

need for the proper neurochemicals. However, the fourth idea—the quality of nerve input received by the brain—changes the whole perspective. A properly working brain is dependent upon receiving nerve signals from joints and muscles that are balanced, reciprocal, and free from noise; anything less than balance is pathology.

> *Neurological motivation requires the means to meet its metabolic demands.*

The joint signals that reach the spinal cord and brain must be free from interference. A healthy brain requires crystal clear signals—static-free if possible, or at least minimal background noise. A static-free joint moves with equilibrium and poise. When the muscles of a stable joint are tested with manual muscle testing procedures, the primary and secondary movers and all of that joint's stabilizers perform as anticipated, according to all that is human.

> *A nociceptor is a sensory receptor that reacts to potentially damaging stimuli by sending nerve signals to the spinal cord and brain. Nociception—the reception of a noxious stimulus—is to the nervous system what inflammation is to immunity. Both are necessary for proper function, but each must be controlled.*

We cannot deny the importance of nutrition in brain function. After all, the constituents of foods provide the foundation for nervous system function. In order for a nerve to carry a signal, the nerve must first be able to change the stimulus into an impulse, and that takes nerve chemicals—nutrients. However, the brain's primary stimulation comes from the nerve signals received and generated from various receptors in the periphery rather than by the presence of nutrients, yet nutrients sustain the brain's neurological performance. It sounds like a circular argument. The peripheral stimulus turns into a nerve signal with the help of biochemicals, and the sustained nerve signals stimulate the brain. Brain stimulation increases its metabolic rate and this requires nutrients that meet the brain's metabolic demands; you cannot have stimulus without sustenance.

Nerve stimulation and nourishment both encourage and prolong neurological longevity wherever they go. The idea is much like conversation at a dinner table. We cannot all talk at once, but a stimulating dis-

> *The terms "strong" and "weak" muscles are schematic for a very complicated neurological process.*

cussion can perpetuate itself and the conversation can last for hours. Conversely, an inappropriate conversation can also be stimulating, but it may not be so orderly. One person may say something that is not received well by another person, causing strife. Another person may say something that leads to an uproar and confusion. The same is true with the human nervous system. When nerve signals travel according to their original programming, the entire nervous system has a pleasant conversation. If, however, the nerve signals take a detour and stimulate areas that should remain quiet or quiets areas that should be stimulated, then abnormal background static erupts and that spawns confusion.

A Tale of Two Hoses

Consider two hoses, each flowing with water. The water from the first hose flows with moderate force while that from the second hose flows powerfully. The first flow represents the signals of nociception and the second flow represents the signals of proprioception—joint motion. The first flow remains constant, but the second flow can vary.

Pretend that these two flows cross in many different places. Now, imagine that the second flow weakens, allowing the first flow a greater opportunity to get through the second flow's path. This example is akin to a joint whose movement is inadequate or lacks the preprogrammed give and take of balance.

Now pretend that the second flow is much stronger. There is no way the first flow could cross that of the second when the second flow is so potent. A robust second flow would block the first flow almost immediately upon contact.

This idea is much like what happens when joint signals break down, and when they are strong and healthy. Joints that are broken down cannot possibly send the right signals to the brain. They lack the competence they once displayed. On the other hand, reciprocal joint signals keep nociceptive signals in check. The nociceptive signals are blocked right where they meet the proprioceptive signals in the back of the spinal cord, forbidding nociception's recognition as pain.

Some aspect of neurological static is always present—it is a product of our physical world. So, in order for the nervous system to work according to its efficient design, we must control or at least minimize static's display. Neurological static can even be related to the production of pain.

No person can ever realistically determine how much pain another person experiences because pain is a private personal experience. Nociception, on the other hand, is the neural process of encoding unconscious pain. Where pain is a conscious experience, nociception is not noticeable until it reaches conscious levels. Only then do we say, "Ouch!" When the nervous system's signals become confused by too much static we realize nociception as pain.

More visibly, neurological static displays itself in abnormal muscle function. When two muscles that support the same joint become imbalanced, joint stability fails and this alters the way the nerves send their signals, and that affects the brain. When muscles test weak when they should be strong and/or stay strong when they should be weak, that's neurologese for, "there is too much nerve static around here!"

Structural problems lead to neurological static, which manifests itself as inflammation and swelling, but it can also show up in your posture and stance, how you rise from a seated posture, and how you walk. Any one, or a combination, of these displays can jeopardize the nervous system's stability and eventually lead to pain. No wonder the brain wants to stop the static! These static patterns can be understood and relieved by a doctor who practices Applied Kinesiology (AK) as functional neurology.

Summary

While the human nervous system is designed to work according to its original plan, in reality that is not often the case; everybody has neurological static. Nutrient imbalances can alter metabolic pathways and abnormal nerve signals can generate unnatural sensory and motor function that leads to abnormal structural responses. The nervous system tends to break down unless it has consistent encouragement to work according to plan. A good doctor can pick up on these abnormal patterns and determine their origin, and will know how to go about fixing them.

Simply providing oxygen to the lungs does not make your body—or the brain—use oxygen properly. Further, eating the right foods, using the right vitamins, or even taking the appropriate drugs does not, in themselves, guarantee any improvement in how the brain works. The brain's environment must remain free of nutritional toxins and neurological static.

The brain also needs to communicate within itself and with all other areas of the body in a coordinated manner. The entire nervous system is capable of keeping all the internal communications coordinated and categorized according to their original design. The trouble comes when these brain systems are unable to speak with one another properly.

Detoxification provides no assurance of tissue health if it falls short of completion. The process of breaking down one large molecule into its component parts needs to work through its metabolic pathways to its natural end. An interruption of the process often leads to harmful offshoots. These offshoots, or unprocessed by-products, often prove more toxic to the system than the original toxin. When these half-processed products remain in the tissues, they perpetuate the havoc.

Finally, the brain needs freedom from static interference. Its signals must be free to work according to their original design for the human nervous system to function optimally. Persistent neurological static leads to brain confusion, which manifests itself in the muscles.

The health of the human brain depends on active metabolic processes. This requires sufficient oxygen and adequate nutrients to keep it going. The brain also needs a clean environment with the ability to communicate within itself and the rest of the body. It also needs crisp, clean incoming and outgoing nerve signals.

The brain's performance is measured by how well it processes its incoming and outgoing signals. When our brain's needs are met—blood, oxygen, glucose, and a specific kind of nerve input and output—our nervous system functions optimally and its tissues remain strong, resilient, and resistant. A properly functioning brain leads to improved health and wellness, as well as a slowed biological clock. This is youthful health.

CHAPTER ONE

RESISTANCE VERSUS ADAPTATION–*THE KEYS TO LONG-TERM WELLNESS*

This chapter will shed some light on the often misunderstood concepts of resistance and adaptation. Although they are often used interchangeably, let us apply two ideas that will distinguish them for all time.

The often misunderstood concepts of resistance and adaptation are important to our understanding of what the brain might say if it could speak because degenerative brain conditions have a gradual onset that comes from both internal and external influences. So far, we have seen that the brain controls all aspects of human function. Eventually, given the right conditions, the brain even affects the incidence of disease. While resistance and adaptation may seem unrelated, they are nonetheless fundamental to how the brain functions.

A healthy tissue is able to resist the stress placed on it by another tissue. Resistant tissues are autonomous, self-sufficient, and self-directed; they are able to function independent of the demands placed on them from elsewhere, like adjacent or physiologically related tissues. On the other hand, adapted tissues undergo a gradual series of worsening changes as they grapple with linked tissues. Such tissues become increasingly unable to keep up with the metabolic demands the breakdown places on them.

Hans Selye, PhD

A Canadian endocrinologist named Hans Selye first used the term "stress" in his book, *The Stress of Life* (1956). Generally, stress relates to the inability of a being or tissue to manage emotional or physical burdens, pressures, or demands, whether actual or imagined.

In the mid-1970s, Selye pointed out that stress is neither good nor bad, but it is how your body *responds* to stress that makes it good or bad. Stress, like energy, makes your body do things; they both generate plastic changes. The body will put stress to use. An appropriate stress response is called *eustress*, while an inappropriate stress response is called *distress*. Where eustress tends to enhance the body's functions, distress tends to systematically take it apart over time, leading to anxiety and general withdrawal.

Richard Lazarus, the late professor in the Department of Psychology at the University of California, Berkeley, de-

---

What Stress Is Not

Contrary to current popular or medical opinion, stress is not:

- Nervous tension. Lower animals and plants have stress, but they have no nervous system.
- The discharge of hormones from the adrenal medulla (the gland that supposedly helps you handle stress).
- That which causes the secretion of adrenal cortical hormones.
- The nonspecific result of damage.
- A deviation from the body's steady state (homeostasis).
- That which causes alarm.
- Identical with the alarm reaction or with the general adaptation syndrome (GAS) as a whole.
- A nonspecific reaction.
- A reaction to a specific stressor.
- Necessarily adverse. It all depends on how it is managed.
- Something that can or should be avoided. Only death truly eliminates a person's stress.

---

fined eustress as exhilarating and innovative; it even enhances the ability to thrive. He said eustress is healthy, giving us a feeling of accomplishment and other positive feelings. Eustress deals with hopeful expectations.

> *The signs and symptoms of distress are, for the most part, all autonomic responses. They represent a fundamental mismanagement of the brain signals that control life-giving processes. Signs and symptoms of distress indicate attempts at adaptation.*

Distress—the tension of breakdown, degradation, or infection—is detrimental. Some particular emotional signs and symptoms of distress may include poor judgment, a generally negative outlook, isolation or depression, excessive worry, oversensitivity, agitation, and even the inability to relax. Distress can lead to dejection, loneliness, and aches and pains. Physiologically, distress can be accompanied by alternating or persistent episodes of diarrhea and/or constipation, nausea, dizziness, chest pain, rapid heartbeat, erratic eating behaviors, inconsistent sleeping patterns, social withdrawal, procrastination or neglect of responsibilities, even addictive behavior (i.e., increased alcohol, nicotine, or drug consumption), and such nervous habits as pacing about, nail-biting, or obsessive-compulsive disorders.

The pursuit of eustress makes one stronger while distress breaks one down. Ideally, if we would all spend more time in the pursuit of eustress, it would overcome distress and health would abound. But as we will see, it is not quite that easy.

General Adaptation Syndrome (GAS)

We may define the General Adaptation Syndrome (GAS) as the manifestation of stress as it develops over time anywhere in the body. Selye's GAS theory described how human tissue—and especially the adrenal glands—respond to stress with alarm, resistance, and

> *The immune system and the nervous system are one in the same system, except that the immune system wanders around the body, while the nervous system remains in place. Whatever is done to one system happens to the other system in the exact same way.*

exhaustion. But stress involves more than just the adrenal glands. Selye also noted that stress involves the stomach, lymphatics, and immune system. He explained that a system subjected to unusual and shocking conditions responds with a countershock reaction—an enhanced retort to overcome the original insult—in an attempt to resist that initial shock phase; but, when the system proves unable to manage the shock, it eventually becomes exhausted.

Just as with any other aspect of life, first we practice in order to learn new things; then we practice to stay proficient at them, and finally we become fatigued by doing the same activities over time and lose our acquired efficiency. The three stages of the GAS are no different. The *alarm stage*, according to Selye, is characterized by an immediate physical reaction, often called the fight-or-flight reaction. Survival is the primary concern, so the system redirects resources from digestive or immune systems to more immediate physiological needs. This leads to an immune system depression with an increased susceptibility to disease.

Resistance is the next of Selye's adaptive stages. As stress levels become more familiar, the system initially kicks up its deterrents to disease, which leads to a false sense of physiological security. However, working at a higher demand level requires increased supplies of the essential materials necessary to maintain this new level of

> *Resistance displays a fundamental ability to perform properly under adversity without burdening other tissues or organs. Adaptation represents a systemic and functional breakdown that taxes other tissues or organs.*

function. Short of meeting the increased metabolic demands, this stage can only last so long and then something has to give.

The *exhaustive stage* described by Selye occurs when the body's systems cannot keep up with the increased demands; the body begins to break down and eventually ceases its efforts to maintain such a high level of stress. Parts of the body literally fall apart and become quite unwell. If significant changes are not made at this point, death may be the result.

Alan Beardall, DC

In the mid-1980s, a chiropractic doctor named Alan Beardall expanded upon Dr. Selye's three stress phases. Just as with Selye, Beardall proposed his own set of relative concepts. He noted a difference between the resistive and adaptive phases. "Resistance," Beardall said, "refers to *the ability* of the inner mechanism of the cell or tissue to perform a task *it was previously unable to achieve without major support from other tissues or organs.*" He then went on to define adaptation as, "*the failure* of the inner mechanism of the cell to perform a task [,] for *it requires support from other tissues or organs.*" Resistance is an intrinsic cellular and/or tissue character that exudes self-sufficiency while it is the nature of adaptation to borrow essential components from the reserves of other tissues or organs.

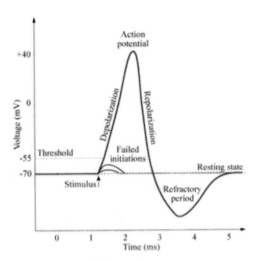

Schematic "Action Potential"

Healthy cells mutually benefit one another; they give and take in order to maintain optimal functional balance. Homeostasis, like the fundamental two phases of a nerve's behavior to either work or be silent, builds on what neurologists call the "all-or-none" theory—a neuron either fires completely or it stays at rest, there is no middle ground.

A "quiet" nerve is said to be at its resting potential (although a nerve always has some level of activity; see *"Failed Initiations"* in the *Schematic "Action Potential,"* above). The resting nerve's activity remains below its level of threshold. But, when the nerve's activity rises to meet that specific threshold, the nerve discharges an impulse. This impulse discharges completely, after which the nerve must take a moment of silence to recharge before it can fire again. This firing of impulses happens all the time in a living system, and each firing stimulates a subsequent nerve in the pathway to the spinal cord and brain. Therefore, as a result of exposure to the stimulus, the nervous system gains greater experience and knowledge—it develops plasticity—about itself and its internal and external environment.

The Effects of Stress

> *Stress is like the sounds around you of which you may or may not be aware.*
>
> *Strain is your response to the stressors around you; you are either consciously or unconsciously aware of them in your environment.*
>
> *Susceptibility is like stepping out of a third-story window—you will not grow those wings.*

Certainly stressors can lead to system troubles that need addressing. Here, the differences between resistance and adaptation become more obvious. When all the essential materials are available to repair the struggling tissues (the Essential Components for Repair, or ECR), the tissues respond according to their original programming. The tissues will always make a physiological decision to maintain its highest level of function in order to survive.

Today's stressors—like yesterday's and tomorrow's—provide a natural stimulus to change. They will both perpetuate life and demand the appropriate homeostatic response or they will drive the nervous system to make calculated decisions it was not designed to manage, making the nervous system an innocent worker in a way contrary to its original programming. This is one of the crimes we unknowingly commit against our brains, letting it slip into compromise without obvious symptoms. At this point, the nervous system probably does not display pain, but it definitely needs help.

If each of the Essential Components for Repair are *Not* Available (ECRNA), Beardall states that the normal body processes are placed "on hold" until all ECRs become

> *Tissue resistance is healthy, but tissue adaptation leads to further compromise and pathology.*

available from either the external or internal environment so that the system can return to normal.

Essential Components for Repair

The external ECRs are thought to be nutritional—carbohydrates, fats, proteins, vitamins, minerals, etc.—energy, rest, exercise, and the absence of negative external factors like financial worries, family problems, infective agents, trauma, overuse syndromes (like exercising beyond your metabolic capacity), etc.

The internal ECRs include such processes of homeostasis as the blood supply, lymphatic drainage, adequate hormones (supplies and/or levels), with a minimal slowing of physiological fluids (like blood, lymph, etc.), and a lack of interference from other systems, like the nervous system. (Section IV of this book deals with a functional nervous system—one that responds in a predictable manner and is free from "static"—which constitutes another internal component for repair.)

Not only must all ECRs be available before an adapted tissue can return to its optimal programming, but these ECRs must exist in sufficient quantities before the body can reestablish wellness. The system that does not make its way back to its original preprogrammed state

Essential Components for Repair (ECRs)

External ECRs	Internal ECRs
Proteins	Blood supply
Carbohydrates	Lymphatic drainage
Fats	Adequate hormones
Vitamins	Minimal stasis
Minerals	Lack of interference, or "static," from other systems, like the nervous system
Energy	
Rest	
Exercise	
Absence of trauma, financial worries, family problems, infective agents, overuse syndromes.	

begins to work in a way that allows its best continuity, but not at its optimal level. We call this a *"functional adaptation with compromise."* That is when, as Beardall said:

1. Some other tissue has taken on at least part of the stressed tissue's workload;

2. This other tissue now takes on altered functions, i.e., stiffness, spasm, hypokinesia, etc.;

3. Somewhere in the body a reduction in performance occurs;

4. The physiological reserve diminishes, draining the body of its abilities to perform according to its original design;

5. The body overall becomes less efficient and more restrictive; and

6. The potential for injury increases.

When the doctor steps in at the right place and time and makes the right diagnosis, and then applies the right therapy, this can influence the healing process toward greater tissue resistance and away from further general adaptation. We want the tissues to resist the negative effects of stress and steer clear of an imbalanced mode. When the body maintains the positive effects of eustress within the restraints of normal endurance, wellness is the result. The ability of such a system to resist stressors of many kinds is at its greatest, and health flourishes. In wellness, all essential components for tissue repair are available; generally, that repair just needs time. Pain plays no part in this phase of health.

Beardall, one of the founding members of the International College of Applied Kinesiology (ICAK), asserted that the level of stress seen when one or any of the ECRs are not available to make the required repairs might be characterized by slight tissue swelling, stiffness, and muscle soreness. If this condition cannot be quickly resolved, the tissues will be forced to take on a different character, called "a holding pattern," until these ECRs do become available. If the ECRs remain unavailable, the tissues move into the acute phase of disease.

The Eight Stages of Adaptation

Stages One and Two

We can say that stage one is when the tissues use the ECRs as needed to work according to their original design. These tissues adapt to stage two when any or all of the ECRs are not available as needed and the tissues get "placed on hold" until the ECRs become available and thus allowing the tissues to revert back to stage one. If the ECRs are not available, then that compromise moves the tissues to stage three. Each of the progressive stages compartmentalizes the involved tissue, but it does not necessarily reflect the state of the person as a whole.

Stage Three: The Acute Stage of Adaptation

The classical symptoms of inflammation—pain, increased temperature, redness, swelling—first appear in the acute stage of adaptation. This occurs when either the ECRs are entirely unavailable to resolve the adaptation or they are available but insufficient in quantities for healing to occur. Time, a very real component of the acute stage, may be exactly what the tissues need to obtain the ECRs and then emerge from the holding pattern set up in stage two. This situation occurs quite commonly during the rehabilitation of bone fractures, ligament strains, cuts and bruises, etc.

Sometimes, the distress on a tissue becomes so great that it needs more nutritional reserves, as may be seen in such conditions as metabolic deficiencies, tiredness, overtraining, worry, etc. If the reserves remain unavailable, the tissues advance to the subacute stage of disease— the first real step into the adaptive

> ### *Applied Kinesiology (AK)*
>
> *The science and art of applied kinesiology is an alternative medical procedure used for diagnosis and determination of therapy. It provides purposeful feedback of the functional state of the body. When used properly, AK assists the doctor in making the right decisions regarding the internal and/or external factors that may be needed for, or are interfering with, the positive changes that would bring about optimal wellness.*

phase. Remember, until this point the tissues have had their needs met to maintain normalcy.

Stage Four: The Subacute Stage of Adaptation

> Beardall states, "...aberrations in the cloacal [i.e., a pelvis centering reflex] mechanism, the gaits, and the group muscles are all physical evidence of the activation of adaptation."

The subacute stage involves more than a holding pattern for struggling tissues, yet it cannot remain here long; this stage is merely transitional. Beardall termed it subacute because of its "tense" conflict. The tissues display a reduced resilience to its situation, yet the symptoms are less involved than the acute stage; the tissue's depletion has progressed just a bit further, but no more damage has occurred yet. He suggested that this is the point in time when the system must commit itself to a definite management strategy of restoration or suffer the consequences of reduced vitality in the injured area.

It must be reiterated here that the goal of any tissue is to survive, but when the tissues cannot rehabilitate and back away from the subacute realm, they will *adapt* their physiology in order to live. Their grip on the tactics that would otherwise bring about resistance wanes and the tissues become generally weaker and more prone to insult. Either the tissue's issues are resolved or the tissues take the next step into long-term illness.

Stage Five: The Chronic Stage of Adaptation

Beardall believed that chronic conditions, while definitely representing a progressed pattern of adaptation, are not usually accompanied by a gross shift in vitality. It is another one of those pain-free crimes we commit against our own brains. People may be dealing with several chronic issues by their fifties. They can experience functional—or what they might consider age-related—compromise, but no overt pain.

The chronic stage is characterized by a reduction in sharp pains because the tissues have undergone a successful adaptation. This is *not* good! The symptoms now range from dull aches, vague sensations, loss of energy, and an inability to perform certain physical feats that may have been possible in the past.

From this chronic stage onward, the tissues "develop coping strategies" to deal with their state of affairs, but this does not necessarily lead to their healing. Just because we no longer feel pain, it does not mean that the problem has gone away. But, if the tissues can obtain the necessary ECRs, the possibility still exists for the tissues to make a U-turn toward a positive resolution. Likewise, if the ECRs remain unavailable, the tissues will degenerate further.

Tissues always endeavor to maintain and prolong their life. Sometimes, however, their local behavior may harm neighboring tissues, challenging those tissues to come up with their own strategies to cope with the added distress. It is like a physiological domino affect; a cascade of failure. Since the function of the whole is greater than the

> *Dr. Beardall once said: "Acute problem in the area stay; chronic problem treat far away."*
>
> *He believed that we should treat acute problems where they are. Moreover, chronic conditions develop "feelers" that seek the support of more peripheral tissues, creating dependency and stress as these tissues intertwine. He taught that greater degrees of tissue resistance are the key to health.*

sum of the function of the individual parts, if these adjacent areas cannot agree on a common strategy to deal with their stress loads, then some local function (or functions) must be sacrificed to maintain homeostasis. Even then the stress will probably be distributed to outlying areas as the system seeks to spread the burden of adaptation more equally, and even this strategy may not benefit the system as a whole.

Stage Six: The Exhaustive Stage of Adaptation

The exhaustive stage tends to be unstable. It appears to be transitional, requiring quick strategic decisions or it will slip further into crisis. At this stage, Beardall states, "...the tissue is metabolically depleted and unable to maintain reasonable energy." Even with rest, this tissue problem will probably not recover. The metabolic pathways that were originally designed to produce the energy can no longer perform to the level required for the maintenance of the tissue's health.

This condition, characterized by a decreasing vitality and function, still falls short of the next stage: degeneration; things get worse.

Stage Seven: The Degenerative Stage of Adaptation

Stages of Adaptation

Selye	Beardall
Alarm	Alarm
Resistance	Resistance
	Acute Stage
	Subacute Stage
	Chronic Stage
Exhaustion	Exhaustive Stage
	Degenerative Stage
	Disintegrative Stage

The ability to revitalize the tissues becomes less likely in this stage. Beardall writes that the ability of the tissues to generate the energy necessary to make meaningful and positive changes takes time to improve and, at this point, time is not in the tissue's favor. "It will take a long time of consistent treatment to allow this area or tissue to regain its vitality. ...Under conscientious treatment, the cells in certain tissues may start modifying and upgrading their function." At this point, hope for healing exists, but it is fading.

The degenerative stage is characterized by an increasing drain on vitality and the development of intensified emotional sensitivity for no apparent reason. The patient may have persistent sleep disturbance, memory loss, significant fatigue, digestive trouble, headaches, joint pain, core instabilities, and circulatory issues. The next phase is disintegration.

Stage Eight: The Disintegrative Stage of Adaptation

In this stage, the will to survive takes over; it becomes the key here, keeping the tissue from dying. The tissue has little to no vitality now because of its degenerative progression; in the tissue's final stage, it becomes ready for death. The person may eat, but they are not really hungry; they may sleep, but only out of exhaustion and it is not rejuvenating. The disintegration may be of a particular tissue, isolated from the body as a whole, and does not necessarily reflect the entire person. However, if nothing is done to surgically remove the disintegrated tissue, the person may die as a result of its presence.

Summary

The conversational line often blurs when people talk about resistance and adaptation. The two are not the same. Resistance keeps a tissue healthy, while conversely, tissues break down because they adapt to their condition; adaptation is not good. Once adaptation sets in, resistance is progressively harder to restore. Resistance maintains the tissue's original function, while adaptation leads to borrowing from and compromising the neighbor's stability until finally both the original tissue and its network have lost their ability to function properly.

The eight stages of adaptation represent the gradual devolution from health to disease; from balance to collapse. The stages may be seen in one tissue, and they could also be within the whole person. The succession from one stage to the next is gradual and is characterized by specific signs and symptoms. The first few stages can be healed with relatively straightforward interventions, but the process becomes increasingly serious as one reaches the last three stages— exhaustion, degeneration, and disintegration.

Dr. Selye was the first to present ideas about his experience with stress, and Dr. Beardall expanded on them in a profound way. While Selye created the general adaptation syndrome, Beardall expanded on Selye's work, applying Selye's theories in a specific way to the human system as a whole. In his private practice and during his years of teaching both applied and clinical kinesiologies, Beardall remained ever mindful of the individual nature of the cells and their metabolic rates as they progressed through time. He stated, "The treating physician [should

> *Resistance and adaptation cannot be interchanged. One is healthy and the other leads to sickness and ultimately death. The former builds depth of function while the latter creates dependency.*

be] concerned about the priorities of the organism and how to help it solve these problems in a reasonable, rational, and natural way if at all possible."

Resistance and adaptation, while often used interchangeably in casual conversation, are not alike. There is a significant difference between them. Resistance describes the cell's ability to function within itself; it does not require the essential components of its neighbors in order to sustain itself. When the stressors placed on these tissues exceed the tissue's resistive resources, there is less ability to resist the event that tends to disrupt normalcy and a greater probability of moving toward adaptation. At first, the stressors have subtle effects, but in the absence of strategies for restoration, the tissues become compromised, which eventually leads to more complicated metabolic compromise.

The doctor's goal is to find ways to help the body build tissue resistance without initiating the adaptive processes. As Beardall reminds us, "Adaptation [that is, alteration of the tissue's metabolic processes away from its original programming] should be a temporary state if the stressors are intense and prolonged. Adaptation leads to tissue exhaustion and death."

Beardall's Eight Stages of Adaptation

Stage	Name	General	Signs	Symptoms
Stage 1	Healthy	Uses ECRs* as needed	Equal give and take of tissue function	Healthy state

(Table continued from page 56)

Stage	Name	General	Signs	Symptoms
Stage 2	Interim	Any or all ECRs are unavailable	Tissues get "placed on hold"	Tissue compromise
Stage 3	Acute	Classic signs of inflamma-tion;	Time is an issue	Metabolic deficien-cies; tiredness; over-training; worry
Stage 4	Sub-acute	A transi-tional stage	Reduced resiliance; resistance wanes;	Tissues progres-sively weaker; more prone to insult
Stage 5	Chronic	No usual shift in vitality; not necessarily painful	Considered "age-relat-ed" compro-mise	Dull aches; vague sensations; loss of energy; inability to perform usual activities of daily living
Stage 6	Exhaus-tive	An unstable stage	[Transi-tional; No specific signs]	Decreased vitality and function
Stage 7	Degen-erative	Revitaliza-tion less likely; time is an adver-sary	Hope for healing still exists, but it is fading	Increased vitality drain; intensified emotional state; persistent sleep dis-turbance; memory loss; signigicant fatigue; digestive trouble; headaches; joint pain; core in-stability; circulatory troubles
Stage 8	Disinte-grative	The will to survive takes over	Eat, but no appetite; sleep, but out of ex-haustion and not rejuvi-nating	Little to no vitality; either the offending tissue is removed or the host dies as a re-sult of its presence.

ECRs=Essential Components for Repair

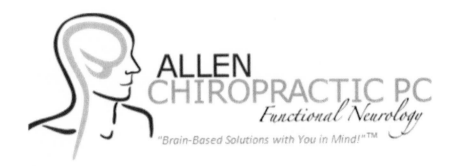

SECTION I

"I CAN'T BREATHE!"

CHAPTER TWO

IF YOUR BRAIN COULD SPEAK, IT MIGHT SAY...

"I Can't Breathe!"

When the brain has trouble breathing, the whole body suffers.

Did you know your brain breathes? All organs breathe. Respiration generates energy, and a byproduct of all energy production is waste. All these toxins must be eliminated or the organs suffer. The lungs and the brain both need their fair share of oxygen, but the brain's breath is not like that of the lungs.

The lungs breathe in oxygen and pass it along to the blood and the rest of the body, while at the same time the blood that returns to the lungs from the rest of the body gives up its wastes—carbon dioxide, CO_2—so the lungs can exhale it

> Oxygen plays a vital role in the breathing processes and in the metabolism of the living organisms.

back into the air. The brain "breathes" too; it is essential for all tissues to change nutrients into energy, including the lungs and brain. The brain's breathing process involves the metabolism of energy by consuming the available nutrients like oxygen, vitamins, minerals, fats, etc., that are found in the brain's blood, and the elimination of its wastes back to the blood. While the lungs breathe oxygen from the outside environment—the air—the brain breathes oxygen from *its* outside environment—the blood. The input and use of nutrients and the elimination of wastes are all essential components to a good, deep breath.

Your brain makes energy so it can put its best nerve signal forward. And your brain uses this energy to produce neurochemicals in response to all the sensory input that reaches the brain. Finally, this energy is necessary to advance the autonomic responses necessary to support movement.

But when your brain gets pushed to exhaustion, what can you do to help your brain catch its breath?

The Breathing Brain

Not everything that happens in the brain has to do with nutrition, but it is biochemical. All the brain's tissues need nourishment, but the neural pathways process their signals biochemically. The brain places top priority on the sensory input it receives from the muscles that create joint motion. While the proper nutrition helps the brain meet the metabolic demands of movement, without joint and muscle input to the brain, human life could not exist. That is, while muscle function places a metabolic demand on the tissues, the human brain also requires sensory input. The nutritional and neurological components are both essential, but the highest priority input for brain function comes from the structure—its muscles and joints.

Joints and muscles send their signals to the brain. That stimulus is what the brain needs to begin its work. All the organs and glands have their own specific controls, of which the brain is the main director, but the brain is different.

Specific types of input stimulate specific receptors. The eyes see, the ears hear, and the tongue tastes, just to name a few. Each type of receptor is specific to the stimulus that it receives. The eyes cannot hear sounds and the ears cannot see the world, but when we hear a loud noise we blink and cover our ears.

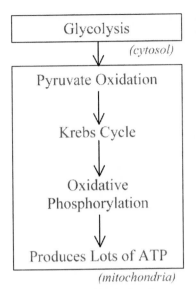

A Summary of the Steps in
Aerobic Respiration

Joint motion, muscle contraction, and nutrition are inseparable. Movement requires muscle function, and muscles require fuel and oxygen that come from nourishment. Healthy joints and muscles depend on available nutrients in order to make neurotransmitters and neurochemicals. These components intermingle as a result of their stimulation—and in the case of nutrition, after it is introduced—the response to which is the indicator of life. Joint stimulation causes the release of neurochemicals in the brain, and neurotransmitters and neurochemicals cause the muscles to contract and joints to move. Each is dependent of the other in their cycles of life.

Before the brain can make neurochemicals, or before the muscles can generate movement, there must be available glucose and oxygen—fuel. This is where nutrition comes in. Both glucose and oxygen are the fuels that make the human nervous system work.

There are more oxygen-sensitive tissues in the brain than in any other part of the body. Any interruption of oxygen, glucose, and/or the system for their delivery to the brain can have detrimental effects on your health, such

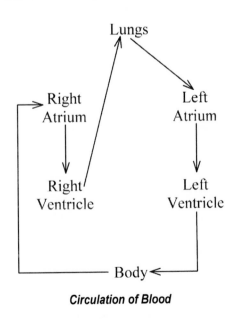

Circulation of Blood

as premature aging or even death. Your brain's delicate functions depend upon a healthy circulatory system, and its delivery of oxygen and a variety of other factors to every neuron in your body.

With every breath, oxygen drenches the blood through the lungs. The oxygen-rich blood's first stop is the heart; from there it takes a high powered ride through the heart, then on to every cell of your body. Most of the inhaled oxygen reaches the brain, whole vessels become progressively tinier until they turn into capillaries that weave in and through the brain and nourish every cell there. Similarly, glucose reaches the neurons via the blood. Capillaries flow close to each neuron—they travel together—and the capillaries nourish the neurons as they travel together.

The average brain accounts for up to 2-3% of the total body mass, yet it requires 25% of all oxygen and 70% of all the glucose used by the body. The kidneys and heart use 12% and 7% of the body's oxygen, respectively. Did you ever wonder why we are so tired after prolonged mental activity? Here is why: At rest, approximately 750ml—25 ounces—of blood is pumped through the brain every minute, and mental activity—like learning—actually increases the brain's oxygen and glucose consumption. That is one of the main reasons why breakfast is the most important meal of the day.

Breathing versus Respiration

Sir Hans Adolf Krebs was a German physician and biochemist. Krebs is best known for his identification of the urea and citric acid cycles. The latter, the key string of metabolic reactions that produces energy inside the cells, is also known as the Krebs cycle, and earned him the 1953 Nobel Prize for Medicine, which he shared with Fritz Lipmann.

All living tissue has a "breath" and this includes the brain. The brain also must breathe. The primary goal of breathing is to take oxygen into and release carbon dioxide from the body. When we say breathing, most people relate to the process of taking air into the lungs and repeatedly and alternately releasing it again in order to stay alive.

Respiration, on the other hand, is more than just moving air in and out of the lungs. It is the physiological process that enables living cells to exchange carbon dioxide, the primary byproduct of cellular metabolism, for oxygen. It is a metabolic process that uses the available nutrients to make ATP and eliminate metabolic wastes. Respiration is the process by which a cell efficiently converts nutrients into useful energy and eliminates the byproducts of that conversion.

Plasticity

The human brain is constantly anticipating ways to change, and it can do so for better or for worse depending upon the brain's metabolic disposition. Brain performance can either improve or it can degenerate. Either way, the brain is changeable and that change can be pain-free. This changeability is called "plasticity"—neuro-plasticity.

Plasticity generally means the ability to be shaped or formed. Brain plasticity relates to learning by either stimulating or inhibiting brain or spinal cord connections of involved pathways throughout the person's life. Just like other brain processes, plasticity uses oxygen and other nutrients to build the connections from one brain cell or local brain center to another. Furthermore, if the necessary oxygen is unavailable, then connections or the tissues go through degenerative changes, without regeneration in most cases. This, too, is considered plasticity, but in a negative way.

While the changing brain is plastic, plasticity is not always good. Adaptation can also be the result of plasticity—negative plasticity—characterized by adaptive changes that can eventually lead to degeneration and disintegration of the system in whole or in part.

Oxygen and Energy

Positive plasticity is functional. Positive plasticity is a result of stimulation that encourages tissues to function for the benefit of the whole system. Positive plasticity is an ongoing cycle of building resistance and eliminating adaptation in the human fabric. Positive plastic changes happen inside the mitochondria and utilize metabolic processes that encourage oxygen to turn fats, carbohydrates, and proteins into energy for healthy tissues.

Anaerobic respiration produces only 2-3 ATP (Adenosine Triphosphate) molecules, in contrast to aerobic respiration, which produces 36 ATP molecules. Anaerobic respiration does not produce a large amount of ATP.

These three basic nutrients can each fuel the Krebs cycle, carbohydrates and proteins yielding four calories of energy, and fats giving up nine calories of energy per gram. (A gram is an internationally recognized unit of measure that assures that the sizes of comparable quantities are identical.)

Generally, the best fuel for the Krebs cycle comes from "healthy fatty acids," like omega 3, 6, and 9 oils—flaxseed, bean, and fish oils—but it can also use both carbohydrates and proteins. Gram for gram, healthy fats burn slowly and yield more than twice the energy found in a gram of either carbohydrate or protein. Refined carbohydrates burn quickly and yield less than half the benefit of healthy fats. The same is generally true for proteins, but proteins contain a nitrogen molecule to deal with, which is the subject for a separate discussion.

Plasticity can only be functional in energy-making tissue that works for the benefit of the system as a whole.

Normally, your brain uses only glucose as a fuel and is totally dependent on the blood for a continuous incoming supply. Interruption of that glucose supply for even brief periods of time (as in a stroke) can lead to irreparable losses in brain function. Your brain uses glucose to carry out ATP synthesis via cel-

There are four calories of energy for every gram of protein and carbohydrate, and nine calories of energy produced for every gram of fat; alcohol produces seven calories of energy.

lular respiration. High rates of ATP production are necessary to maintain a healthy nerve membrane, keeping it responsive to essential stimulation. When the nerve cell's membrane becomes tired, its resting level tends to drift progressively closer to threshold (recall the Schematic "Action Potential", diagram above) until it finally discharges abnormally, sending a signal when it should be silent; this is called a *spontaneous discharge*.

Your brain turns that glucose into a special kind of fuel called ATP, which is produced via the Krebs cycle in the mitochondria of every cell in your body. Simply illustrated, during the aerobic—oxygen dependent—metabolism of the six carbon glucose molecule into three two-carbon molecules called pyruvic acid, there should be two molecules of ATP, then another two molecules of ATP for every completion of the Krebs cycle and finally another thirty-two molecules of ATP at the end of the electron transport chain—thirty-six molecules of ATP for every molecule of pyruvic acid (see "the Pathways of ATP Production" below).

Placing a healthy metabolic demand on any cell makes it work with greater efficiency. This is especially true of brain cells. Remember that efficient tissues have a resistance that is not available to tissues that are tired—or adapted. Unless a cell's metabolic demands are met by making its essential components for repair readily available, metabolic compromise leads to a vicious cycle of an adapted functional state and further metabolic compromise.

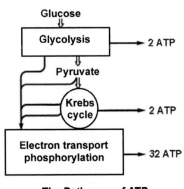

The Pathways of ATP Production

Because of their unique nature that requires plenty of oxygen, there can be as little as a few or several hundred of these "breaths" happening in the mitochondria of every brain cell. This creates an abundance of available energy. However, when the stimulation to the brain's cells fades away because the structure is broken down and sending fewer signals, the demand on the mitochondria withers and the cells develop trouble breathing; the available oxygen and glucose is less than adequate and the brain's cells "gasp for breath." This is called hypoxia—inadequate oxygen reaching the body's tissues. Even mild hypoxia—a functionally anaerobic condition—can be damaging. Remember that the Krebs cycle is aerobic, and if the brain's

Recall that a healthy neuron rests far from the threshold of excitation. All the aspects of healthy metabolism keep the cell membrane quiet until it needs to fire, and then it does so completely and then it rests. A cell that is anaerobic, for example, is unhealthy and its resting level tends to drift toward the threshold level requiring less stimulation before it can fire. In fact, a sick nerve can fire for practically no reason at all, even discharging itself, causing things to happen that should not be happening, and vice versa.

metabolic demands ebb with a resultant reduction in the available oxygen—hypoxia or functional anaerobics—the mitochondria produce only two molecules of ATP instead of the usual thirty-six. That leads to cellular metabolic compromise and overall brain exhaustion. If the demand on the brain continues, but the brain has a reduced ability to perform useful work, even for short periods, then the brain's abilities dwindle as its metabolic capacity falls behind its functional demand.

Even mild hypoxia hampers complex learning tasks and reduces short-term memory. It also hinders subconscious learning. Tasks that require no conscious involvement, such as muscle contraction and balance, also suffer during hypoxia. If we allow cells to remain in an oxygen-starved gasping-for-breath state, this may lead to thinking problems and impaired motor control. This is our brain's way of saying, "Something has to change because I cannot catch my breath!"

Symptoms of hypoxia show up in the body, including bluish skin (cyanosis) and an increased heart rate. Prolonged oxygen deprivation results in fainting, long-term

Remember that too much or not enough of any substance can create disease.

loss of consciousness, coma, seizures, cessation of brain stem reflexes, and eventual brain death.

Before we run off in the direction of "more oxygen, more oxygen," too much oxygen or its inappropriate use can have its drawbacks. For example, when you cut an apple and leave it out, it turns brown similar to the way new bicycle spokes eventually rust. These are

Fats—lipids—consist of numerous chemical compounds that are insoluble in water but soluble in organic solvents. Lipid compounds are of many different types, but we can call them fatty acids. Dietary fats supply energy, carry fat-soluble vitamins (A, D, E, K, and F), and are a source of antioxidants and bioactive compounds. Fats are also incorporated as structural components of the brain and cell membranes.

examples of slow oxidation—the gradual interaction of oxygen molecules with other substances. The quick ignition of dry grass in a field is an example of *fast* oxidation. In general, both slow and fast oxidation lead to the breakdown of whatever it is with which they react. Oxidation is important for the conversion of one substance into another, but its benefits must be controlled by antioxidants. Conversely, too few antioxidants lead to the presence of "free radicals," which are *unstable* and very corrosive bits of oxygen.

Free radicals can react very quickly to link different molecules together so they can be "stable" again. Unfortunately, these links are often unnatural, leading to molecular combinations that can damage cell membranes. This is especially damaging to the fatty parts of those cell membranes of brain nerves because of their high affinity for oxygen.

Summary

Once stress crosses the precarious line from a state of resistance into the cascade of adaptation, radical oxygen atoms increase their toll. Some theories suggest that aging is no more than the amassing of damage caused by free radicals, which is distressing to tissues. Keeping free radicals under control—the domain of antioxidants—is one of the biggest keys to long-term brain health. So, if we want to stay young, then we need to breathe right, manage our sugars, keep moving, and keep our free radicals at a minimum. Now that is a sensible anti-aging program!

CHAPTER THREE

TEACH YOUR BRAIN
TO BREATHE BETTER

If your brain could speak, it might say, "I'm tired!"

Having a healthy brain—feeling your best, being mentally focused, energetic, and balanced—is the result of how you treat it. What foods you eat, the exercise you do, and the sleep you receive all contribute to building a better brain.

> *Free radicals are essential for many functional metabolic reactions, so their presence and their involvement must be controlled with antioxidants, not quenched by taking too many of them.*

And the verdict is in: We are not treating our brains well.

Today, brain problems manifest themselves as tiredness and lack of focus, but they also display themselves in all major brain disorders. Sadly, two-thirds of Americans are obese and ninety-seven million have pre-diabetes, and both of these conditions wreak havoc on the brain, increasing the risk of depression and dementia.

Our brains respond to use; the more you use your brain the stronger it becomes. And just as with physical exercise, the benefits of "mental exercise" depend on your brain's ability to breathe.

Scientists at one time believed that the brain's circuitry was fully linked by adolescence and impossible to change in adulthood. However, today we know that every brain has the very high possibility of staying plastic well into old age. Best of all, this research has opened up an exciting world of possibilities for functional neurological treatments for head trauma, strokes, and many other injuries—even warding off Alzheimer's disease.

> *I remember seeing an experiment using mouse traps and ping pong balls. The traps covered the room's floor. They were set side-by-side with ping pong balls set on the traps. Everything was stable until the researcher tossed in one ping pong ball. Imagine what happened. That free ping pong ball hit the first trap, setting off a chain reaction with a barrage of ping pong balls until all the traps were fired. The same mechanism happens with free radicals when they are uncontrolled by antioxidants.*

Free Radicals

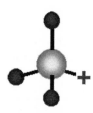

A Free Carbon Radical (represented by the "+" sign)

There is much talk lately about free radicals. Do you know what free radicals are and why they can be harmful? They are like fire that can both help and hurt you.

Free radicals are high energy molecules created when oxygen interacts with certain unprotected molecules leaving an atom, or groups of atoms, with an odd (unpaired) and highly unstable number of electrons. Free radicals play a favorable role in the pathways of glucose metabolism to ATP. Every millisecond of every day of our lives the natural metabolism of blood glucose to ATP generates free radicals.

Free radicals come from various aspects of everyday life, like food additives, harmful smoke, smog, pesticides, infections, fried and barbecued foods, and alcohol. They are also formed in your skin by excessive ex-

A Free Carbon Radical (represented by the "•" sign)

posure to the UV component of the sun's radiation. That is why the skin of those living in hot climates tends to age earlier. Apart from those generated by your body's own biochemistry, free radicals are also present in car emissions and other pollutants such as ultraviolet light,

> *Electrons generally travel in pairs, and when one of that pair is lost through a chemical reaction, the other electron has only one purpose in its short life: to pair up with another electron and it will do whatever it has to do in order to achieve that. It is called a free radical, and its life is short.*

detergents, agricultural chemicals, and many other sources.

> *Free radicals are what make us look older as we age: they destroy skin cells as they form, yet that is one of the least of their effects. They can also oxidize low density lipoproteins (LDL) that carry cholesterol throughout your body, which theoretically leads to plaque on the walls of your arteries. This is a common theory for the serious cardiovascular condition known as atherosclerosis.*

While free radicals are essential to many natural processes, once formed, and when uncontrolled, the mission of these highly reactive militant molecules is to capture or share an additional electron in order to become stable again—and their stability is not necessarily a healthy thing. Free radical reactions can be so intense that they can start a chain reaction, like dominoes falling one after another; one free radical violently snags an electron from another molecule and so forth, leaving nothing but unhealthy molecular combinations in their wake.

The chief danger posed by free radicals is the oxidation or corrosion they create in vital cellular components, from the peripheral cell membrane to carbohydrates, lipids, and most importantly the DNA at the cell's core. Free radicals can make fatty parts of cells function poorly or even destroy body cells—having a dramatic effect, both visually on your skin, and internally on your

> *Phytonutrients, phytochemicals, zoonutrients and zoochemicals all contain non-food nutrients that enhance how other biochemicals work. They have a positive effect on metabolic changes.*

general health—if they get a chance. To prevent free radical damage the body has a defense system of *antioxidants*.

The Cellular Membrane

Anthocyanins impart a red to purple coloration.

The membrane of every cell is made up of three layers—two layers of protein and one layer of fat, or "lipids." In fact, both the brain that we see and its microscopic parts—the nerves and their connections that link everything together to create and maintain memories—are primarily made of fats, making them extremely susceptible to free radical attack; free radicals love fats. Antioxidants protect against fat breakdown by neutralizing free radicals and lessening the severity of their attack.

Certain foods are an excellent source of antioxidants. One very good way to control the free radical population is to consume lots of fresh, organic fruits and vegetables—include plenty of color in your diet.

The clutter that causes memory loss like Alzheimer's disease may be sorted out by eating berries—specifically blueberries, strawberries and acai berries, either frozen or fresh.

Eat Your Vegetables

Most vegetables can be eaten raw, making them taste just as vivid as their color. Carrots, celery, squashes, and corn are delicious raw. It is commonly thought that root vegetables need to be cooked before they are eaten, but that is not necessarily true. The flavor of the raw root vegetables can vary depending on where they were grown. Raw turnips, for example, may be more tender and delicate, and others more crunchy, hence their reputation that they need to be cooked. Several different radishes, rutabagas, and grated beets are de-

The most heat labile vitamins (those sensitive to temperature changes) are ascorbic acid, thiamin, vitamin D and pantothenic acid. Further, when heated, vitamin B6 and pantothenic acid are significantly reduced by 67 and 62 percent, respectively.

licious raw. Fresh summer turnips are often sweet, moist, and crispy when raw.

Train Your Brain

> Nature uses the least amount of everything.

If your brain could speak, it might say, "I need your help!" Teach your brain to enjoy foods in their raw state, thereby "training the brain." Start out slow by eating raw carrots and peas that can be very sweet and crunchy, which tackles two basic needs. Then, gradually take on more of an advanced curriculum with raw turnips and the like.

Fresh raw fruits and vegetables contain the nutrient antioxidants, Vitamins A, C, and E, and the mineral antioxidants copper, zinc, and selenium. However, other dietary food compounds, such as the *phytonutrients* in plants and the *zoonutrients* in animal products, are thought to have greater antioxidant effects than either vitamins or minerals. These are called non-nutrient antioxidants and include *phytochemicals*, such as lycopene found in tomatoes, and anthocyanin found in cranberries.

> Known vitamin complexes are biologically and inextricably linked with individual minerals to form a functional molecule. If you supplement your diet with a distilled vitamin fragment and/or an individual mineral, you do not have a complexed vitamin even if you consume the vitamin's parts all at the same time.

It takes a variety of different nutrients to keep free radicals under control and nerve cell membranes protected. Antioxidants are special molecules that can safely interact with free radicals. They keep an eye out for potentially dangerous chain reactions before vital molecules are damaged.

Vitamin and Mineral Complexes

Vitamins and minerals are essential for the growth and function of the brain. And while nature holds many mysteries, there is one that is revealed here: vitamins and minerals always work together as a whole unit. You cannot fractionate a vitamin from its associated mineral and still have the original natural substance; separating a vitamin from its associated mineral splits a biochemical— "bio" means "life" —into mere chemicals. Nature couples vitamins and minerals for a reason and they should stay that way until they are metabolized by the body.

> *A deficiency of the essential components for repair places undue stress on a tissue's delicate balance. In response, that tissue's function adapts and gets placed on hold until the required nutrient(s) become available.*

Although several enzyme systems constantly scan for free radicals, the principle micronutrient (vitamin) antioxidants are the Vitamin A, Vitamin C, and Vitamin E complexes. They each play an important role by helping electrons and two-carbon organic groups safely transit each cell's metabolic pathways.

> *Carrots are the most common example of a food that is rich in Vitamin A Complex. A "complex" vitamin is a whole substance made up of many synergistic parts. The most familiar form of Vitamin A (beta-carotene) does not contain the whole "Vitamin A Complex" as it is found in nature.*

Unchecked free radicals can lead to cellular breakdown. They can change the metabolic nature of the entire cell, especially affecting the fat-soluble molecules, oxidizing or corroding the cell membrane. Free radicals accelerate the aging process and increase the likelihood of more serious neurological problems such as psychosis, Alzheimer's disease, certain cancers, atherosclerosis, cardiovascular diseases, cataracts, age-related macular degeneration, immune dysfunction, rheumatoid arthritis, and movement disorders like Parkinson's disease.

Vitamin A Complex

The molecule commonly known as Vitamin A complex is an oil-soluble antioxidant that, as far as we know, contains four of the 563 identified carotenoids—the most common one being beta-carotene—as well as the minerals magnesium, manganese, and zinc.

Vitamin A complex acts as a *gate keeper* to control the size of the membrane's openings that allow certain substances into and out of the cell. It also acts as a *flow meter* to control the flow at which fluids and/or essential components for cellular repair pass through these membranous channels.

Vitamin A complex helps hold cells together; it regulates the cell's membrane integrity. Vitamin A strengthens the cilia (minute hair-like structures)

Margarine also contains vitamin A, but margarine is not a food. It has no nutrient value; nothing will grow on it. By virtue of its configuration, margarine should be considered unfit for human consumption! It should properly be found in the non-food section of your supermarket—that part in the center of the store with all the preservatives, additives, colorings, and the trash can liners—because its structure is one molecule different from that of plastic.

found in the trachea, lungs, and fallopian tubes. These cilia prevent entry of foreign particles, pathogens, and microorganisms into the body. When it comes to breathing, cilia are essential for proper ventilation. Even the brain has cilia that act as a sensory organelle to receive signals that regulate cellular behavior and physiology.

Research suggests that diets rich in berries can reduce, or even reverse, declining brain function. Blueberries, in particular, have been shown to have the ability to improve memory and keep your brain "young." They can also help improve your balance and coordination.

Berries are rich in antioxidants that protect your brain cells from oxidation and free radical damage. This means antioxidants may slow down brain aging and prevent disease, while promoting the growth of healthy brain cells. Berries are also some of the most colorful foods you can eat!

List of Healthiest Berries:

Acai berries	*Boysenberries*	*Mulberries*
Blackberries	*Cranberries*	*Raspberries*
Blueberries	*Gogi berries*	*Strawberries*

A deficiency of Vitamin A complex causes the cell membrane to become sloppy. The channel size widens, allowing the wrong substances to gain entry, or keeping the essential components normally contained inside the cell from erroneously escaping, contributing to the cell's toxicity. For example, sodium is normally found in the fluid outside the cell, only gaining access to the cell's interior under certain circumstances. However, if the sodium channels become inefficient and allow too much sodium into the cell at the wrong time, it changes the cell's electrolyte concentration gradients. Since water always follows sodium, the interior of the cell tends to swell leading to a very good probability that the cell's nucleus will be displaced and the cell's membrane will rupture, resulting in the cell's instant death. Adequate Vitamin A complex can help avoid such a catastrophe.

Vitamin A complex is also important in cellular immunity, gene transcription, embryonic development and reproduction, bone metabolism, the making of red blood cell components, and skin and cellular health. It is also important in good vision, and the growth and maturity of white blood cells.

Vitamin A complex can be found in carrots, liver, fish-liver oil, green leafy vegetables, egg yolks, milk products, and yellow fruits.

Vitamin C Complex

Vitamin C, as nature intended, occurs biologically in its complex form. It is a water-soluble antioxidant compound that has been used to protect the body against oxidative stress, and is a cofactor in several vital enzymatic reactions.

> *Vitamin P (citrin) maintains the resistance of cell and capillary walls to permeation and is effective in treating purpura (skin hemorrhages).*

It contains ascorbic acid, as well as Vitamins P, J, and K, rutin, hesperidin, and bioflavonoids. The Vitamin C complex also includes several other important factors, including copper—an antioxidant mineral—which is bound to the amino acid tyrosine, creating an enzyme called tyrosinase. By itself, Vitamin C—ascorbic acid—is just a chemical. The Vitamin C complex is not the same as ascorbic acid, the chemical compound commonly marketed as "Vitamin C." However, in its tyrosinase-containing state, the Vitamin C complex becomes a biologically active nutrient.

Vitamin C complex is part of the ground substance matrix—the non-cellular components that contain the fibers. Collagen is not usually considered part of the ground substance, but it does include all the other large complex, often chain-like, organic molecules that contain carbon, hydrogen, oxygen, nitrogen, and usually sulfur, and, most prevalent, water. Think of it as composing the background that holds cells in place, the way mortar holds bricks in place to make a solid wall—but a solid wall of immune strength. The ground substance matrix is amorphous, almost gel-like, and provides structural cellular support in addition to performing various other important functions. A deficiency of the Vitamin C complex causes the cells and the tissues they compose to become sloppy, opening them up to immune problems.

The Boomerang Effect: Taking mega dose vitamins over a long period of time can lead right back to the signs and symptoms of the disease for which the original vitamins were taken to combat.

A rich source of Vitamin C complex is found in fruits like rose hips (the fruit of the rose plant), acerola, black currant, guava, kiwifruit, papaya, strawberry, orange, lemon, grapefruit, raspberry, and lime; and in vegetables like red pepper, parsley, broccoli, Brussels sprouts, cauliflower, garlic, spinach, and cabbage. It is also found in certain cuts of meat, especially liver, but many believe that today's liver contains too many toxins to be beneficial.

The vast majority of plants and animals are able to formulate their own Vitamin C complex through a sequence of four enzyme-driven steps that convert glucose to Vitamin C complex. Human cells, however, are unable to make their own Vitamin C complex, therefore it must be consumed. The *whole Vitamin C complex* is an essential nutrient for humans, making it an important metabolic key for healthy tissues.

Vitamin E Complex

Vitamin E complex is probably the best known of all the oil soluble antioxidants and free radical scavengers. It occurs naturally in some foods and is added to others, and it is available as a dietary supplement.

The actual collective name for its eight different known oil soluble factors is the Vitamin E complex—intimately connected to the antioxidant minerals chromium and sele-

> *Consuming distilled or fractionated vitamins can set off a cascade of peripheral nutrient stress that starts in the local tissue and invades the healthy tissue, breaking down their natural resistive nature and leading to adaptation and beyond.*

nium, as well as the tocopherols, tannins, phospholipids, and other organic nutrients—each part having its own unique aspect of biological activity. They are all found naturally in the same molecule, and if you take each of these components separately, they work less efficiently—even pharmaceutically—than if they were left together. The eight different Vitamin E factors work synergistically to protect the cell membrane from the damaging effects of oxygen free radicals and peroxides. Without having all eight factors together, complete with their natural cofactors, Vitamin E is just another distilled and fractionated chemical.

It used to be thought that one needed a lot of Vitamin E (d-alpha tocopherol) in order to protect sensitive tissues from free radicals. Most health experts used to recommend that their heart patients take up to 1600 international units (IU) of Vitamin E per day with minimal side effects. However, we now know that too much distilled Vitamin E can be toxic to the tissues, leading to an increased mortality *and the incidence of heart failure* in patients with chronic diseases.

> *No two people require the same form, dose, or frequency of vitamins. Each person is unique and so are their nutrient requirements.*

To control some of the fervor, the Food and Nutrition Board of the National Academy of Sciences (2000) specified the Recommended Dietary Allowance (RDA) of Vitamin E as 15 IU per day, and listed the Tolerable Upper intake Level (UL) of any alpha-tocopherol form as 1,000 IU per day. The UL is the upper level that is *likely to pose no risk of adverse health effects* to almost all people in the general population. Today, even using 1,000 IU per day is considered to be too high. However, Vitamin E toxicity has rarely been documented in humans.

Vitamin E complex can be found in avocados, almonds, hazelnuts, sunflower seeds, spinach, other green leafy vegetables and their cold processed oils, and wheat germ. It can also be found in whole grain foods, milk, eggs, and asparagus. Vitamin E complex is stored in adipose tissue or body fat, liver, and muscle.

More about
the Essential Components for Repair

Foods High in Vitamin A & C Complexes
• *Mangos*
• *Oranges*
• *Carrots*
• *Broccoli*
• *Tomatoes*
• *Cantaloupe*
• *Rainbow chard*
• *Red, Green & Yellow peppers*

In theory, taking only the individual parts of vitamin complexes—i.e., beta-carotene as Vitamin A, ascorbic acid as Vitamin C, or d-alpha tocopherol as Vitamin E—leads to tissue depletion. Over time, the depleted tissues start attracting the missing essential components necessary for their repair from nearby tissues, making the deficient tissues whole again. This sets off a spreading domino effect that starts in the local tissue and invades deeper and more peripherally into the healthier tissues, breaking down their natural resistive nature. This cascade eventually leads to the process of adaptation, which gradually leads to more manifest disease.

Working with ACEs

The Vitamin A, C, and E complexes are powerful micronutrients with antioxidant qualities that promote and preserve memory in the elderly. These three vitamin complexes are thought of as the most common antioxidant vitamins.

It is commonly known that these complexes provide the best defense against the damaging effects of free radicals. It is also well known that brain tissues are very vulnerable to oxidation. However, it is not so readily known that these three vitamin complexes easily cross the blood-brain barrier, making them essential to a healthy brain. The ability to cross the blood-brain barrier makes these three vitamin complexes readily available to do their work of protecting the brain tissues from oxidation.

Misplaced Antioxidant: Vitamin B Complex

The Vitamin B complex has a very special protective effect on nutrients, and it is for that reason that it is included here. The Vitamin B complex is a group of water-soluble nutrients that coexist in the same foods and play a vital role in cellular metabolism.

The Vitamin B complex is particularly important for proper function of—and energy production in—the nervous system, and is perhaps the most important nutritional factor for healthy nerve cells. As a whole, the Vitamin B complex helps the nerves produce energy as well as manage stress, anxiety, tiredness, irritability, headaches, and asthma.

Vegetables and fruits also contain natural sugars that aid alertness. Your brain needs natural sugars to function at its best.

Avocados are rich in good fat and vitamin E, while whole and sprouted grains are rich in fiber. Both are good for your circulation. And what's good for your blood flow is great for your brain.

The B complex supports and increases the metabolic rate of every cell. They are an essential component of the Krebs cycle. Certain Vitamin B complex cofactors are involved in moving the metabolism of one glucose molecule into a cascade of metabolites for the ultimate purpose of making ATP. The B complex also helps to maintain healthy skin, increase muscle tone, enhance immune and nervous system function, and promotes cell growth and division—including that of the red blood cells that help prevent anemia. Finally, the B complex also helps carry oxygen to the brain and helps eliminate damaging free radicals—thereby supporting neurotransmitters like acetylcholine, and sharpening both the memory and the senses.

The individual Vitamin B fractions are never found alone in their natural form, although they are often referenced individually. When the several parts of the Vitamin B complex are distilled or fractionated into the more commonly known independent factors—like B1, B2, B3, B5 (pantothenic acid), B6, B9 (folic acid or folate), B12, etc.—they behave more like chemicals than whole food nutrients. However, the B-vitamins are more powerful when they are consumed in their naturally bound or complexed form. Because of their synergistic effects, taking the entire B complex in its whole and naturally bound form is always healthier than taking the individual factors by themselves.

Vitamin companies love to increase the individual B component potencies to what is considered the recommended daily allowance (the RDA) for the vitamin fractions. However, the RDAs are unnecessary when using vitamins in their complex form—whole foods—because nature would never use such large potencies by themselves. In fact, the more concentrated potencies may even be detrimental to the cell or tissue's vital processes.

Taking the Vitamin B components individually may aid certain well known body processes, just as scientific literature claims. But when consumed over a long period, their overall benefit eventually leads to undesirable secondary peripheral effects similar to those found with any other distilled or fractionated substance, such as drugs or pharmaceuticals. An individual B-vitamin may have a scientific benefit, but when they are separated from the whole complex they act more like drugs than nutrients. Their effectiveness is seldom equal to that found in whole foods. They may work quickly, but they cannot work better than the whole complex in the long run. To prevent the inevitable side effects, nature actually binds these Vitamin B factors into one complex unit that also contains zinc, cobalt, and many other trace nutrients.

The B-vitamins are some of the most commonly mega-dosed supplements, making the urine of people taking them bright yellow, indicating the presence of expensive urine. This reaction is considered normal, but the individualized products place undue stress on the eliminative organs—the liver and kidneys, for example. In fact, taking individual and high potency B-vitamins for long periods of time can lead to the need to supplement with other substances to subdue the side effects brought on by the use of products that are picked apart or separated into their individual components. This includes vitamins, minerals, and even certain drugs. There is no way around it: these dissected products are synthetics to body tissues because they are no longer in their complex form.

While these three antioxidant vitamins—A complex, C complex, and E complex—and the B complex may be some of the most common, there is another group of nutrients that we can also add to our arsenal in the war on free radicals: the minerals. Minerals are the brick and mortar aspects that help build tissue resistance.

Minerals

> *Tissue mineral levels are influenced by other tissue nutrients like fats, carbohydrates, proteins, and even other minerals.*

Many different minerals are needed in order for the body to function properly, and many are needed in very small amounts. They act as catalysts or coenzymes—"helper molecules"—that in turn activate enzymes or proteins, which control the thousands of biochemical processes occurring in the body in several different biochemical reactions. They enter a metabolic process to cause a certain reaction, and then leave the reaction having done their job.

In fact, each vitamin complex knits a particular mineral at its center; some vitamins contain more than one mineral. Vitamin A complex encases magnesium, manganese, and zinc. Further, the B12 (cyano-

> *Chlorophyll is a complex molecule that gives green vegetables their color. It holds magnesium at its center.*

cobalamin) fraction of the Vitamin B complex, for example, contains cobalt as its fundamental mineral. Another essential part to this molecule that helps the red blood cell carry oxygen is heme, which contains iron.

There are at least fifteen minerals that are essential to health. Either inadequate or excessive dietary intake of any or all of them can lead to mental and behavioral problems, including depression, often before any physical symptoms appear.

Magnesium is one of the great alkaline minerals. It balances brain chemistry and builds strong bones. It has a profoundly positive effect on the small blood vessels, which helps the heart and keeps it beating steadily. Magnesium also helps keep blood sugar levels stable and blood pressure levels healthy. It is also essential for the metabolism of calcium from bone and for the normal metabolism of the energy used by the pumps that manage the flow of sodium and potassium ions across the cell membrane, so important in keeping cells healthy. If these pumps become crossed up, the cell can quickly take on too much water causing it to burst.

Magnesium is said to be the most deficient major mineral in the Standard American Diet, with over 80% of Americans chronically deficient. Simply processing whole wheat or brown rice into bleached white flour and bleached white rice—by refining out and processing the magnesium-rich wheat germ and bran—depletes over 75% of the magnesium.

One of the best food sources of magnesium is Cacao—healthy chocolate; *Theobroma cacao*, the cocoa tree. Eating a wide variety of legumes (beans and peas), nuts and seeds; whole, unrefined grains; spinach and other green vegetables will help you meet your daily dietary need for magnesium.

Finally, while not advocating its consumption, tap water can be a source of magnesium, but the amount varies according to the water supply. Water that naturally contains more minerals is described as "hard." There is more magnesium in "hard" water than there is in "soft" water.

Manganese is quite important for normal blood and nerve function. It is found in trace amounts in the bones, liver, kidneys, and pancreas—usually in its natural, organic,

> *Manganese is necessary for the metabolism of Vitamin B1 and Vitamin E.*

and crystalline bound forms. Manganese is an essential trace mineral of connective tissue, bones, blood clotting factors, and sex hormones. It also helps metabolize fats and carbohydrates, and aids in calcium absorption.

Low levels of manganese can contribute to infertility, bone malformation, weakness, and seizures. While it is considered fairly easy to consume enough manganese in your diet, some experts estimate

> *Drinking water provides many different minerals, but that does not make it a good source of minerals.*

that as many as 37% of Americans do not get the recommended dietary intake (RDI) of manganese in their diet.

> *Fingernails can tell a lot about a person's long term health.*

Good sources of manganese are nuts and seeds, wheat germ and whole grains (including unrefined cereals, bulgur wheat, and oats), buckwheat, legumes, and pineapples. The American diet tends to contain more nutrition-depleted refined grains than whole grains, and refined grains only provide half the amount of manganese as whole grains.

However, too much manganese in the diet could lead to high levels of manganese in the body tissues, including the brain, and that is not good. Too much manganese can be associated with poor cognitive performance in school children, and when too much makes its way into the basal ganglia, it can lead to neurological disorders similar to Parkinson's disease.

Zinc is another trace mineral, involved in more than three hundred enzyme systems that help heal wounds, maintain fertility in adults and growth in children, help protein synthesis, and influence cellular reproduction. It is needed for a strong immune system, healthy cell division, and protection against free radical damage. Zinc, together with magnesium and manganese, is an integral part of the Vitamin A complex, having the ability to enhance the transport of Vitamin A from the liver. Good sources of zinc include oysters, meat, eggs, seafood, black-eyed peas, tofu, and wheat germ.

The signs of a zinc deficiency might include white spots or bands under your fingernails, fatigue, diarrhea, and a reduced sense of taste or smell. Fish oil supplements are a good alternative to zinc supplements because they contain zinc in addition to other essential vitamins and minerals, and their fatty animal proteins promote your body's zinc absorption.

Common Fingernail Complaints and Possible Remedies

Deficiency Symptoms	Possible Nutrient Need	Contributing Factors
Soft, tear or peel easily, opaque white lines	Protein; Calcium	Stomach pH issues; fatty acid need
Dry, brittle, break easily	Protein; Calcium	Stomach pH issues; fatty acid need
Horizontal lines, grooves or ridges	Protein; Calcium	Stomach pH issues; fatty acid need; too rigorous manicuring; poor nutrition habits; recent illness or surgery
Vertical lines, grooves or ridges	Calcium metabolism	More apparent with age; possible hypothyroidism
Small white spots or bands on nails or in nail bed	Zinc; Vitamin A complex	Possible nail base injury, 2-3 months earlier; possible liver/kidney disease; a consequence of fasting or menstruation
Thin, flat, concave (spoon-like) shape, yellow nail beds or white coloration near the cuticle with dark coloration near the tip of the nail	Vitamin A complex; Vitamin E complex; Iron; Iodine	Possible chronic liver/kidney disease; iron deficiency and/or thyroid malfunction

(Table continued from page 85)

Deficiency Symptoms	Possible Nutrient Need	Contributing Factors
Yellow nail bed, poor or no growth	Vitamin E complex	Possible lymphatic or respiratory congestion; diabetes, lung disease, psoriasis, fungal infection, overuse of nail polish
Darkened nail beds	Vitamin B complex	Need for greater circulation in the smallest vessels
Extra-large or missing half-moons	Thyroid nutrients	Hypo- or hyperthyroid
Very round club shaped	Vitamin B complex	Congenital heart or lung disease
Brittleness	Vitamin A complex	Exposure to too much water and soap, or dehydration

As important as zinc is, overdosing can be a serious problem. While zinc aids metabolism, too much zinc actually hinders the absorption of many other vitamins necessary for tissue health, cancelling out even the wisest food choices and their benefits. Specifically, too much zinc will affect iron, copper, and magnesium. Zinc toxicity also lowers your body's immunity and good cholesterol levels.

Potassium is essential for the proper function of all cells, tissues, and organs in the human body, especially of the heart, kidneys, muscles, nerves, and digestive system. It is also an electrolyte, a substance that conducts electricity in the body. Sodium, chloride, calcium, and magnesium are also electrolytes. The right potassium balance in the body is relative to the amount of sodium and magnesium in the blood. Usually the food you eat supplies all of the potassium you need.

Good sources of potassium include citrus juices (such as orange juice), bananas, avocados, cantaloupes, tomatoes, potatoes, lima beans; and fish like flounder, halibut, salmon, cod; and chicken and other meats.

Certain diseases (kidney disease and gastrointestinal disease with vomiting and diarrhea) and drugs, especially diuretics ("water pills"), remove potassium from the body. Diarrhea, vomiting, excessive

> The misuse of diuretics can lead to depression because they can deplete essential mineral levels.

sweating, malnutrition, and malabsorption syndromes (such as Crohn's disease) can also cause potassium deficiency. Potassium can be supplemented to replace potassium losses and prevent potassium deficiency.

Having too much potassium in the blood—common in Western diets that use a lot of salt—is called hyperkalemia; too little is known as hypokalemia.

Sodium is essential for normal body function. It helps to regulate blood pressure and blood volume, and it is critical for the proper function of muscles and nerves.

The most common form of sodium is sodium chloride, which is common table salt, although salt and sodium are not the same things. Sodium occurs naturally in most foods. Milk, beets, and celery also contain naturally occurring sodium, as does drinking water, although the amount varies depending on the source.

Many people are unaware that "hidden" sodium found in processed foods (as salt) makes up the largest proportion of the sodium consumed by adults (in addition to any personally added salt). Processed meats, such as bacon, sausage, ham, and canned soups and vegetables are all examples of foods that contain added sodium. Fast foods are generally very high in sodium.

Sodium is also added to various food products in various forms, such as monosodium glutamate (also known as MSG), sodium nitrite, sodium saccharin, baking soda (i.e., sodium bicarbonate), and sodium benzoate. These additives are common to condiments and seasonings such as Worcestershire sauce, soy sauce, onion salt, garlic salt, and bouillon cubes.

Since water follows sodium, too much sodium—hypernatremia—can lead to high blood pressure in sensitive people, and a serious build-up of fluid in people with congestive heart failure, cirrhosis, or kidney disease. Such people should be on a strict sodium-restricted diet, as prescribed by their doctor.

Both calcium and magnesium are involved in numerous metabolic functions and are absolutely essential for the maintenance of a healthy body. Calcium is considered the backbone mineral because of its role in the formation of skeleton and teeth. Magnesium is called the natural tranquilizer due to its relaxing action on nerves and muscles.

In addition to high blood pressure or hypertension, increased heart attack risk, stroke, and kidney failure are all well-known side effects of an increased daily intake of salt. The medical costs of treating these, and other conditions related to excessive table salt intake, also take a serious toll on our collective pocketbooks.

Potassium and Sodium are considered together because they help determine the body's electrolyte balance, which regulates water levels. Eating a lot of salty food (sodium)

Deficiencies or excesses of certain minerals may impair brain function.

disrupts this balance. This not only produces high blood pressure, but also affects neurotransmitter levels, producing depression and premenstrual syndrome in women. In addition, the misuse of diuretics, or "water pills," can lead to potassium deficiency, which in turn can manifest itself as depression.

Calcium works with magnesium to maintain balance, or homeostasis, in the body, much as sodium and potassium work together to achieve balance in water levels. If you are supplementing with calcium, you will need to take one-half as much magnesium as calcium, sometimes even more, to keep the two properly balanced. This includes women who are taking calcium supplements to prevent osteoporosis.

Depressed individuals often have excessive calcium levels, particularly those with bipolar disorder. When these patients

> *While minerals are essential to the body, they don't provide energy.*

recover, their calcium levels usually return to normal. Depression can also occur in cases of calcium deficiency, long before the appearance of physical deficiency symptoms.

Chromium is a trace mineral said to have no verified biological role in human nutrition. However, trace amounts of chromium do play a role in sugar and lipid metabolism. It protects against fatty deposits on the walls of blood vessels and is useful in HDL cholesterol in men. Nearly 80% of Americans are deficient in chromium.

Mineral deficiencies can be attributed to these factors:

- *Starvation*
- *Poor diet*
- *Poor absorption of vitamins and minerals*
- *Damage to the digestive system*
- *Infection*
- *Alcoholism*

In larger amounts, chromium can be toxic; in fact, it can be carcinogenic. In its picolinate form, chromium can produce chromosomal changes in hamster cells (use caution when giving chromium to your hamster as a supplement).

Chromium is widely distributed in the food supply, but most foods provide only small amounts. Meat and whole-grain products, as well as some fruits, vegetables, and spices are relatively good sources of chromium. In contrast, foods high in simple sugars (like sucrose and fructose, as in high-fructose corn syrup) are low in chromium.

Selenium is one of the most important trace minerals to human physiology. It works as an antioxidant, playing an important role in maintaining the health and proper function of your immune system and thyroid.

The content of selenium in food depends on the selenium content of the soil where plants are grown and animals are raised. Human selenium deficiency is rare in the United States, but it is more common in other countries, most notably China. A deficiency may contribute to a form of heart disease, hypothyroidism, and a weakened immune system. There is also evidence that selenium deficiency alone does not usually cause illness. Rather, it can cause the slow adaptation that eventually leads to the increased susceptibility to illnesses caused by other nutritional, biochemical or infectious stresses.

Selenium can be obtained in a variety of foods including liver, butter, garlic, and whole grains. Fish and seafood are also good sources of selenium, specifically, mackerel, herring, flounder, oysters, scallops, and lobster. Other potential sources include Brazil nuts and sunflower seeds. Plant foods are the major dietary sources of selenium in most countries throughout the world.

High blood levels of selenium can result in a condition called selenosis. Symptoms of selenosis include gastrointestinal upsets, hair loss, white blotchy nails, garlic breath odor, fatigue, irritability, and mild nerve damage.

Copper is an essential trace element mineral that serves a wide variety of purposes within the body, both on its own and as a cofactor, meaning it is a vital part of chemical processes that involve other vitamins, minerals, other nutrients or other substances. Although the body requires a comparatively tiny amount of copper per day, even that little bit is crucial to optimum health and performance. Human organs with the highest copper concentrations are kidney and liver, followed by brain, heart, and bone in decreasing order. Copper helps metabolize oxygen in cooperation with iron.

A copper deficiency can occur in people who supplement with zinc without also increasing copper intake. Zinc interferes with copper absorption. A deficiency can also be related to an iron deficiency anemia, as well as blood vessel ruptures, bone and joint problems, frequent infections, loss of hair and skin color, fatigue and weakness, difficulty breathing, irregular heartbeat, and skin sores.

Excessive intake of copper can cause abdominal pain and cramps, nausea, diarrhea, vomiting, and liver damage. In addition, some experts believe that elevated copper levels, especially when zinc levels are also low, may be a contributing factor in many medical conditions including schizophrenia, hypertension, stuttering, autism, fatigue, muscle and joint pain, headaches, childhood hyperactivity, depression, insomnia, senility, and premenstrual syndrome. Although copper toxicity does not normally happen in humans, too much copper is a contributing factor in Wilson's disease.

Excellent food sources of copper include asparagus, turnip greens, blackstrap molasses, calf's liver, and crimini mushrooms.

Sources of Antioxidants

Good sources of antioxidants include:

- *Allium sulphur compounds: leeks, onions, and garlic.*
- *Anthocyanins: eggplant, grapes, and berries.*
- *Beta-carotene: pumpkin, mangos, apricots, carrots, spinach, and parsley.*
- *Catechins: red wine and tea.*
- *Copper: seafood, lean meat, milk, and nuts.*
- *Cryptoxanthins: red capsicum, pumpkin, and mangos.*
- *Flavonoids: tea, green tea, citrus fruits, red wine, onion, and apples.*
- *Indoles: cruciferous vegetables such as broccoli, cabbage, and cauliflower.*
- *Isoflavonoids: soybeans, tofu, lentils, peas, and milk.*
- *Lignans: sesame seeds, bran, whole grains, and vegetables.*
- *Lutein: leafy greens like spinach, and corn.*
- *Lycopene: tomatoes, pink grapefruit, and watermelon.*
- *Manganese: seafood, lean meat, milk, and nuts.*
- *Polyphenols: thyme and oregano.*
- *Selenium: seafood, lean meat and whole grains.*
- *Vitamin C: oranges, black currants, kiwifruit, mangos, broccoli, spinach, capsicum, and strawberries.*
- *Vitamin E: vegetable oils (such as wheat germ oil), avocados, nuts, seeds, and whole grains.*
- *Zinc: seafood, lean meat, milk, and nuts.*
- *Zoochemicals (i.e., health-promoting compounds found in animal foods.): red meat and fish. Also derived from the plants animals eat.*

Iron is considered an essential trace mineral. It helps carry oxygen throughout the body and helps us to convert food into energy. It helps the blood carry oxygen to the brain; therefore, it is believed to improve concentration and intellect and may increase the attention span.

Many foods contain iron, such as brown rice, whole wheat, wheat germ, oatmeal, raisins, sunflower seeds, soy, broccoli, green beans, lima beans, beets, peas, dates, prunes, blackstrap molasses, and many others.

Iron deficiency is the most common nutritional deficiency and the leading cause of anemia in the United States. Iron plays a key role with many enzymes that help digest foods, and is required in numerous cell functions. When our bodies do not have enough iron, various parts of our bodies are affected.

On the other hand, excessive iron can lead to toxicity, especially in men, since they do not lose blood as women do through menstruation. Therefore, men

> *Vitamins and minerals are essential to the body but are not manufactured by the body. Hence, these materials must be consumed within our daily diet.*

should not supplement with iron unless under a doctor's direction. Too much iron is called hemochromatosis; an iron overload. It can have genetic and non-genetic causes. Early signs and symptoms of hereditary hemochromatosis mimic those of many other common conditions, making it difficult to diagnose. Signs and symptoms of hereditary hemochromatosis include joint pain, fatigue, loss of sex drive (libido) or impotence, lack of normal menstruation (amenorrhea), and pain on the upper right portion of the abdomen.

Cobalt is the most potent mineral known to man, and it is essential for all animals. It is found in most common foods, and is readily absorbed by the gastrointestinal tract. Cobalt is at the center of the most common cobalamin, Vitamin B12, which is the primary biological reservoir of cobalt, uniquely making it an "ultra-trace" mineral.

> *Herbs have long been used to enhance brain performance. Some people believe that herbs help improve memory, enhance mental abilities, increase concentration, raise mental alertness, and increase attention spans.*

Although cobalt needs are met in a well-balanced diet, the precise daily intake requirement is not known, and cobalt deficiency in humans has not been seen.

Cobalt, like all other metals, becomes toxic at excessive levels and leads to many harmful and potentially permanent side effects, like cardiomyopathy, hypothyroidism, and neurological damage, as well as impairing the senses. Excess cobalt can cause neuropathy, seizures, blindness, headaches, and liver damage. Cobalt toxicity has also been linked to cancer. After nickel and chromium, cobalt is a major cause of contact dermatitis.

<u>Boron</u> may be an essential trace mineral for animals and humans. It protects the cell from neutron radiation damage and DNA strand breaks, which can lead to neuronal death, creating an enhanced risk of memory loss. Boronated compounds have been shown to be potent anti-osteoporotic, anti-inflammatory, hypolipemic, anti-coagulant, and anti-neoplastic agents both *in vitro* and *in vivo* in animals. Not enough research has been done with boron supplements to determine their safety and side effects.

Herbs that Enhance Brain Function

Herbs and brain function share a long relationship. Herbs profoundly influence many brain functions. Herbs are thought to improve memory, boost mental aptitudes, enhance attentiveness, increase mental awareness, and benefit attention spans.

Herbs primarily improve circulation, providing a greater presence of oxygen and other nutrients that brain cells need to generate more fuel. They also act as antioxidants

> *The half-life of phytonutrients may vary from several hours to several days.*

to protect nerve cells by preventing them from being damaged by free radicals. Antioxidants are also proven cancer fighters. And finally, they recharge neurotransmitters such as serotonin, dopamine, and norepinephrine, which regulate feelings, thoughts, and memories.

Herbs are an excellent example of substances that contain vitamins, minerals, and phytonutrients in their naturally-bound and complex forms; herbs are whole foods. They provide both the essential components for tissue repair and the whole nutrients to help the tissues endure the stresses placed on them by the demands of daily living.

> *The term adaptogen is used by herbalists to refer to a natural herb product that is proposed to increase the body's resistance to stress, trauma, anxiety and fatigue. All adaptogens contain antioxidants, but antioxidants are not necessarily adaptogens, and their antioxidant qualities are not proposed to be their primary mode of action.*

One of the beneficial aspects of brain-based herbs is their flavonoid content. Flavonoids are found in the deep red and blue pigments of fruits, wine, and teas. They protect against oxidation and the harmful effects of sunlight.

The number of beneficial brain herbs is too great to cover here, and continued research is finding more applications for them every day. However, here are several of the better known herbs that have proven themselves helpful in particular brain conditions.

Of all the organs, the brain is the single largest consumer of oxygen, and Gingko biloba is one of the best-known bioflavonoid-containing memory herbs. Gingko works primarily by dilating the blood vessels and increasing the oxygen in the blood that eventually reaches the brain. This makes Gingko an excellent supplement for people as they age, since aging generally reduces the oxygen-carrying blood flow to the brain contributing to memory loss.

> *Although it is commonly considered ginseng, Siberian ginseng cannot currently be marketed as "ginseng," since the term "ginseng" is reserved for the Panax species.*

Gingko increases adenosine triphosphate (ATP; the valuable end-product of the Krebs cycle) levels in the tissues and acts as a free radical scavenger. Ginkgo also increases acetylcholine levels, allowing efficient transmission of the body's electrical impulses.

Ginkgo acts as an antioxidant, protecting brain cells against damage from free radicals that may contribute to Alzheimer's disease and dementia as people age.

Ginkgo side effects and cautions include: possible increased risk of bleeding, diarrhea, gastrointestinal discomfort, nausea, vomiting, headaches, dizziness, heart palpitations, and restlessness. If any side effects are experienced, consumption should be stopped immediately.

Ginseng has been said to benefit the understanding. Ginseng is a root herb that has been used in China for thousands of years, and in America since the 1700s to restore alertness and improve memory. It grows in Korea, Russia, and America, but each variety has a slightly different characteristic and their quality varies greatly.

All ginseng acts as an "adaptogen"—they help the body cope with all kinds of physical and psychological stress. While *Panax ginseng* (the genus and species names for Asian ginseng) is the most popular form used today, Siberian ginseng is the one that is most often included in products geared to improve cognitive ability, but the Siberian ginseng is not the same as other ginsengs. Both ginsengs are in the same family, but the Siberian ginseng has a different genus (*Eleutherococcus* as opposed to *Panax*). So if cognition is the goal, use the *Eleuthero* form of ginseng.

There appears to be some evidence that ginseng also benefits the brain. A recent Chinese study found that a ginseng compound improved the memory in scores of people suffering from stroke-induced dementia. People generally break their ginseng into small pieces and chew it as a common energy booster, and it is a familiar ingredient in many energy drinks. It is also believed to support the immune system.

As far as the brain is concerned, ginseng's power appears to come from its ability to control and lower the release of the stress hormone cortisol, which is deadly to the brain. People who use ginseng appear to have greater accuracy, speedier response times, increased mental and physical stamina, and have improved their standard cognitive function scores by an average of more than 50% on some tests. Ginseng appears to improve the quality of life and reduce episodes of depression in women.

Results from a recent study indicate that by concentrating some of ginseng's active ingredients— those substances either unknown or that may require cofactors in order to achieve therapeutic goals—

> *Herbs contain many of the life-giving nutrients essential for proper brain function, some known and others unknown.*

it could protect rats from the effects of a toxin designed to mimic the degenerative process seen in Huntington's disease (severely impaired movement and loss of neurons). Further studies believe that the rat model could also be relevant to other degenerative diseases, such as Parkinson's disease.

> *Herbs, in general, should not be used by women who are pregnant, or nursing. Always contact your doctor before using herbs if you are not familiar with their properties.*

Ginseng's side effects can include nausea, diarrhea, headaches, nosebleeds, high and/or low blood pressure, and breast pain. One of ginseng's most common side effects is the inability to sleep. However, other sources state that ginseng causes no sleep difficulties, so it is quite possible that its effects are individualized. Ginseng may also induce mania in depressed patients who mix it with antidepressants.

Gotu kola is known as an adaptogen; it is one of the most vital rejuvenating herbs available. It is an Asian herb that has been used for generations to improve mental function and treat a host of aliments from wounds to insomnia. It stimulates the brain and fights fatigue by combating stress and bringing about more restful sleep—thereby counteracting the effects of sleep deprivation, reducing anxiety, and increasing clarity of thought. Gotu kola helps improve circulatory problems (venous insufficiency) including varicose veins, and blood clots in the legs, it can heal trauma, and reduce some types of high blood pressure. It also helps increase memory and intelligence.

Gotu kola contains certain chemicals that seem to decrease inflammation in the vessels and blood pressure in the veins. Gotu kola also seems to increase collagen production, which is important for wound healing. It has few side effects and interactions.

Sage is another brain-oriented herbal supplement. It is an outstanding memory enhancer, having been found to aid in word recall; it strengthens the nervous system, improves memory, and sharpens the senses. The reason for this is unclear, but researchers believe that it may be because sage increases the levels of certain neurochemicals.

Sage has one of the longest histories of use of any medicinal herb. When taken orally, it is commonly used to improve cognitive function in people with Alzheimer's disease. Early research shows that sage may also aid hypoglycemia.

The leaves and stems of the sage plant contain antioxidant enzymes, including SOD (superoxide dismutase) and peroxidase. Sage has been said to have a unique capacity for stabilizing

and preventing oxygen-based damage to the cells.

Rosemary helps stimulate the immune system, increase circulation, and improve digestion. Rosemary is a good source of the minerals iron and calcium, as well as dietary fiber, and it contains Vitamin B6. It also contains anti-inflammatory compounds that have been shown to increase the blood flow to the head and brain, improving concentration.

Rosemary has been commonly used as a circulatory and heart stimulant, and has had a long lived reputation for improving memory. It has been shown to have possible antioxidant properties perhaps related to its carnosic acid, which has been found to possibly shield the brain from free radicals, lowering the risk of strokes and neurodegenerative diseases like Alzheimer's disease and Lou Gehrig's disease. Rosemary may help stimulate the memory, strengthen mental clarity, and relieve mental fatigue, helping recall.

Muscle and joint pain and the symptoms of gout have been relieved throughout history with rosemary, and its oil is sometimes used to treat muscle pain and arthritis.

Saint John's wort (also known as Tipton's Weed or Klamath Weed) can both fight depression and strengthen the immune system. It is most widely known for its positive influence on anxiety and tension; it acts as an antidepressant. It appears to be equally as effective and have fewer side effects than

> *Please use Saint John's wort "sensibly." It may significantly alter the therapeutic, absorption, metabolism, and/or toxic effects of many prescription and non-prescription drugs.*

standard antidepressants. St. John's wort can be especially useful in treating the depression related to chronic fatigue syndrome and systemic candidiasis; both are related to immune dysfunction.

Studies have shown that Saint John's wort extracts may exert their antidepressant actions by inhibiting the re-uptake of the neurotransmitters serotonin, norepinephrine, and dopamine. It is also useful in treating swollen veins since it contains the bioflavonoids that generally serve to improve venous-wall integrity and reduce vascular fragility and inflammation.

Passionflower is used to ease sleep problems, gastrointestinal upset related to anxiety or nervousness, and generalized anxiety disorder. Passionflower is believed to reduce palpitations, irregular heartbeat, high blood pressure, fibromyalgia, pain relief, and improve overall systemic mood and function.

> *As with most other herbs, people with asthma and hay fever should use herbs with caution, as herbs have been found to aggravate these conditions in susceptible people.*

The chemicals in passionflower have calming, sleep inducing, and muscle spasm relieving effects. It has also been used in cases of Attention Deficit Hyperactivity Disorder (ADHD), and it may help reduce or prevent insomnia.

Passionflower can cause side effects such as nausea, dizziness, vomiting, confusion, irregular muscle action and coordination, altered consciousness, and inflamed blood vessels, and more rarely arrhythmia and palpations. It should be used only under supervision.

Oatstraw is good for nourishment and rejuvenation. It benefits pain relief, calms and strengthens the nervous system, relieves stress, strain and overwork, calms emotions, fights anxiety and panic attacks, boosts immune function, and it reduces depression and nervous exhaustion. It improves coordination, strengthens digestion, helps stabilize blood sugar, soothes headaches, encourages deep restful sleep, and nourishes the heart, circulation and endocrine system. It enhances clear thinking and improves attention span, showing a benefit for hyperactive children and the elderly.

Oatstraw is an excellent source of calcium, iron, phosphorous, and B-vitamins, but it is slow acting. Depending upon the person, the desired response may require several doses over a week or so. Oatstraw has been used in herbalist traditions for hundreds of years. No drug interactions or side effects have ever been reported.

While there are no known drug or nutrient interactions associated with the use of oatstraw, please note that if you are allergic to oat flour it may be a good idea to avoid any products containing oatstraw. Because oatstraw contains gluten, those suffering from Celiac disease should avoid it in any form.

Skullcap helps calm the nerves with its anti-spasmodic and sedative qualities. It is helpful in the treatment of epilepsy, hysteria, anxiety, and delirium tremens. Skullcap can also be used to induce sleep naturally without the negative effects of many prescription and over-the-counter sleep aids. It is becoming better known as an alternative treatment of attention deficit disorder (ADD/ADHD), and it is sometimes used to treat the symptoms associated with anorexia nervosa, fibromyalgia, and even mild Tourette's syndrome.

Overdose symptoms include giddiness, stupor, confusion, irregular heartbeat, and twitching. There have been no documented cases of negative interactions with other herbs or medications. However, skullcap does have a sedative effect and should not be combined with prescription sedatives.

Rose hips is said to be a medicine for the heart and body. The anti-inflammatory properties of rose hips have recently been shown to be useful in the treatment of patients suffering from knee or hip osteoarthritis. It could be more effective than pain medications for easing the pain of arthritis sufferers. The pain-relieving properties of rose hips—which have previously been linked to reduced inflammation in osteoarthritis—have been suggested for decades. In numerous studies, rose hips was almost three times more effective than standard acetaminophen—a widely used over-the-counter analgesic (pain reliever) and antipyretic (fever reducer)—at relieving pain. It was also almost 40% more effective than another common therapy, glucosamine. Rose hips powder also did not have the side effects associated with other pain medications, including constipation and drowsiness.

A natural source of Vitamin C, rose hips has been touted as a useful laxative, capillary strengthener, and a boost to the immune system to prevent illness. It contains significant Vitamin C, tannins, pectins, and carotene (carotenoids, including beta-carotene), lycopene, lutein, and a few other phytonutrients. Although Vitamin C has been studied extensively for its effects, studies on rose hips are lacking.

Some herbal references claim that the leaves have been used as a poultice to heal wounds. The rose hips are useful in the treatment of influenza-like infections, diarrhea, and various urinary tract disorders. No side effects are known when rose hips are used in the normal designated amounts.

"Phytofoods" are foods that come from plant-based sources. "Phytochemicals" emphasize the plant source of most of these protective, disease-preventing compounds. "Phytonutrients" better describes the compound's "quasi-nutrient" status. "Nutraceuticals" are specific chemical compounds found in foods that may prevent disease. "Functional foods" are those foods that, by any other name, would taste as good.

Chamomile has anti-allergenic, anti-inflammatory, anti-diuretic, anti-spasmodic, sedative, and anti-tumor properties, with the oil having anti-bacterial properties as well. Chamomile's anti-inflammatory properties make it a good choice for rheumatoid arthritis sufferers, osteoarthritis or other painful swelling disorders. Its anti-spasmodic effects make it useful in treating spasms and cramping, including menstrual cramps. Chamomile is often used to treat nervous disorders such as insomnia, anxiety, and nervous tension. It is also used internally to treat spasms and inflammation of the digestive tract.

This herb is safe for use in children and may help with children's problems that have a nervous component. However, chamomile has been shown to cause allergic reactions to people who have allergies to other members of this daisy-like plant family (of the family Asteraceae, including arnica, artemisia, feverfew, tansy, and yarrow). People on blood-thinners such as Coumadin® or Warfarin® should consult their physician before using chamomile because it may enhance the effects of the medications.

The New Technology of Phytonutrients

Phytonutrients, (*phyto-* is Greek for plant) are essential plant-based nutrients. The particular components may or may not be known—they may have a name, or have yet to be discovered; phytonutrition is an evolving field. Nevertheless,

> *Phytonutrients are not considered essential for life, but they are significant in maintaining a healthier life of better quality.*

phytonutrients are considered to be those life-giving essences that are the difference between a food that is living and one that is lifeless. This is the same idea as we previously discussed with complex vitamins.

Lately, there has been more and more written about phytonutrients and their role in our health. Many nutritionists and their patients are becoming more familiar with phytonutrients and their importance in the antioxidant picture. These foods are not new, but science has added newer understanding to the benefits these foods deliver and how we can obtain them.

For example, a new company has recently developed a breakthrough substance to treat radiation sickness based on phytonutrient activity. The company reports that the natural character worked better than the pharmaceuticals, which used to be the doctor's first choice.

How Phytonutrients Protect Our Health

* *Serve as antioxidants*
* *Enhance immune response*
* *Enhance cell-to-cell communication*
* *Alter estrogen metabolism*
* *Convert to vitamin A (beta-carotene is metabolized to vitamin A)*
* *Cause cancer cells to die (apoptosis)*
* *Repair DNA damage caused by smoking and other toxic exposures*
* *Detoxify carcinogens through the activation of the cytocrome P450 and phase II enzyme systems*

Phytonutrients are living components that come from plants, and are thought to promote health. Recent research has indicated that phytonutrients can be divided into classes on the basis of similar protective functions, and their individual physical and chemical molecular characteristics. They are complex molecules, many with hard to pronounce names—such as carotenoids, including lycopene, as well as flavonoids, phytates, isothiocyanates, lignans, phenols, saponins, and many others. High amounts can be obtained from fruits and vegetables that have strong colors. They are also found in grains, legumes, and nuts. Teas are also rich sources of phytonutrients. One of the well-known phytonutrients is lycopene, found in tomatoes.

The phytonutrients are believed to contribute to human health. While not specifically classified as nutrients that are essential for survival, phytonutrients do contain elements that can help promote good health. Because they often contain antioxidants and compounds that are anti-inflammatory in nature, phytochemical foods are sometimes known by the nickname "superfoods."

Apart from the major food principals like protein, carbohydrates, and fats, a large number of food items we consume consist of invaluable plant-derived

When it comes to wise food purchases, people are learning to stay away from foods whose labels contain words they cannot pronounce. In the case of phytonutrients, more education is the difference between buying and avoiding.

chemical substances. There are over 10,000 known phytonutrients, and their antioxidative effects boost the immune system. They are anti-inflammatory, antiviral, antibacterial, and provide cellular repair. Although their caloric value is insignificant, consuming adequate levels of phytonutrients is crucial since their potential benefits of health promotion and disease prevention are enormous.

Phytonutrients contain important cofactors—or "helper molecules"—that many times have been processed out of manufactured (or "manufractured") foods. They are enzyme-like factors that are quite heat sensitive, making them susceptible to the methods of food preparation. Often, when the temperature of a phytonutrient-rich food reaches body temperature—37°C or 98.6°F—the phytonutrients break apart leaving only inactivated remnants that have no nutritional benefit. The solution is to eat most of your food raw.

A healthy diet consists of about 85% raw food, and the other 15% can be cooked. Of course, raw meat, poultry, and seafood should always be avoided. There are lots of unhealthy consequences from eating uncooked animal products.

While phytonutrients are not considered to be the essential nutrients of life, they are thought to be excellent sources for the care and maintenance of a healthy body and mind. Choosing to include at least a few of the fruits, vegetables, and spices that contain these impor-

Foods with Specific Color

- *Red: tomatoes, watermelons, cranberries*
- *Red-Purple: grapes, cherries, strawberries, blackberries, pomegranates, endive, olives*
- *Orange: squashes, mangos, carrots, pumpkin, cheese, kumquats*
- *Orange-Yellow: oranges, pineapples, apricots, cantaloupe, mangos, lemons, papayas, yams*
- *Yellow-Green: avocados, spinach, green beans*
- *Green: broccoli, cabbage, cauliflower, watercress, spinach, asparagus, apples, beans, tea*
- *Blue: blueberries, bilberries, blue potatoes, blue corn*
- *Purple: eggplant, plums, prunes, figs, grapes, cabbage, carrots*

tant elements in the daily diet will prove helpful in maintaining both physical and mental wellbeing.

Here are a few of the more common phytonutrients and some of the ideas about how they work.

Carotenoids are a component of the Vitamin A complex, generally protecting your cells from the damaging effects of free radicals. Carotenoids represent one of the most widespread groups of naturally occurring pigments. These compounds are largely responsible for the red, yellow, and orange color of fruits and vegetables, and are also found in many dark green vegetables. They enhance the performance of the immune system and help the reproductive system to function properly.

In addition to their antioxidant and immune-enhancing activity, carotenoids have shown the ability to stimulate cell-to-cell communication. It is now believed that poor communication between cells may be one of the causes of cellular overgrowth, a condition that eventually leads to cancer. By promoting proper communication between cells, carotenoids may play a role in cancer prevention.

Food sources of carotenoids include carrots, sweet potatoes, spinach, kale, collard greens, papaya, bell peppers, and tomatoes. To maximize the availability of the carotenoids in the foods listed above, these foods should be eaten raw or lightly steamed.

High intake of carotenoid-containing foods or supplements is not associated with any toxic side effects. However, one indicative sign of excessive consumption of beta-carotene is a yellowish discoloration of the palms of the hands and soles of the feet. This condition is called carotenodermia (a yellow-orange discoloration of the skin), and is reversible and harmless.

Lycopene is not an essential nutrient for humans. However, it is commonly found in the human diet, mainly in dishes prepared from tomatoes. It is absorbed relatively easily from the stomach and transported in the blood by various lipoproteins to accumulate in the liver, adrenal glands, lungs, prostate, colon, and testes. While lycopene is chemically a carotene, it has no Vitamin A activity.

Lycopene is a bright red carotenoid pigment and phytochemical found in tomatoes and many other red fruits and vegetables, such as red carrots, watermelons and papayas, pink guava, sea-buckthorn, goji (a berry relative of tomato), asparagus, dried parsley, basil, and rose hips. Although they too are red, strawberries and cherries contain no lycopene. Excessive consumption of lycopene can cause a deep orange discoloration of the skin. Like carotenodermia, lycopenodermia is harmless.

> *Oxidative reactions are like a pilot light in your cells. Your water heater and gas stove, for example, have a pilot light. It is a flame that stands ready; it constantly burns. Under the right circumstances—upon demand—it can cause a greater flame meant for good. But when that pilot light gets out of control, it can ignite an entire city block.*

Lycopene is fat-soluble, so oil is said to help its absorption. You might think that cooking tomatoes would reduce the bioavailability of lycopene, but it actually becomes concentrated. Cooking and crushing tomatoes (as in the canning process) and serving in oil-rich dishes (such as spaghetti sauce or pizza) greatly increases lycopene's assimilation from the digestive tract into the bloodstream.

Processed tomato products such as pasteurized tomato juice, soup, sauce, and ketchup appear to contain the highest concentrations of bioavailable lycopene from tomato-based sources. In fact, the lycopene found in tomato paste is four times more bioavailable than in fresh tomatoes. That is why tomato sauce is a preferable source of lycopene as opposed to raw tomatoes.

A literature search appears to indicate no well-established definition of "lycopene deficiency," and direct evidence supporting the repletion of low lycopene levels is lacking. However, there are cases of intolerance or allergic reaction to dietary lycopene, which may cause diarrhea, nausea, stomach pain or cramps, gas, vomiting, and loss of appetite.

Flavonoids used to be known as Vitamin P, probably because they are a vascular—or capillary—permeability factor, but this term is rarely used today. Nonetheless, as discussed earlier, they are an intimate part of the Vitamin C complex.

Flavonoids are readily available in a wide variety of foods, and they have a relatively low toxicity compared to other active plant compounds. Therefore, many animals, including humans, ingest significant quantities of flavonoids in their diet. Flavonoids appear to be quite efficient fighters of a wide variety of free radicals.

Like all antioxidants, the health benefits of flavonoids are based on their ability to reduce the damage caused by free radicals. There are a number of different flavonoids that can provide antioxidant power to your body. These include catechin, kaempferol, quercetin, xanthohumol, epicatechin, myricertin, and epigallocatechin. In addition, flavonoids in particular are said to have amazing health properties, including anti-bacterial, anti-diarrheal, and anti-viral effects. Flavonoids can help reduce allergic reactions, and may even shrink tumors and improve vasodilation.

You can increase your flavonoid, antioxidant, and essential vitamin levels by simply eating more fruits and vegetables. Strawberries, blueberries, spinach, and onions are good flavonoid sources. Other robust flavonoid sources include tea—green, black or white—and honey.

Lignans are a group of biochemical compounds found in plants and act as antioxidants and insoluble fibers. Some debate exists whether lignan-rich foods play a role in the prevention of hormone-associated osteoporosis, cancers, and cardiovascular diseases. There is some evidence that they are capable of binding to estrogen receptors, which allow them to interrupt the cancer-promoting effects of estrogen on breast and endometrial tissue while at the same time promoting anti-inflammatory proper-

> *There are two general categories of foods that have been associated with disrupted thyroid hormone production in humans: soybean-related foods and cruciferous vegetables. In addition, there are a few other foods not included in these categories—such as peaches, strawberries and millet—that also contain goitrogens.*

ties that protect or suppress cancerous changes, mainly defending against heart disease and colon cancer.

Their main sources are fruits (particularly strawberries and apricots), legumes, and whole grains, such as rye, wheat, oat and barley—rye being the richest source—and seeds, such as pumpkin, sunflower, poppy, and sesame, but flax seed and sesame seed contain higher levels of lignans than most other foods. However, lignans are not associated with the oils that come from foods, so flaxseed oil does not typically provide lignans unless ground flaxseed has been added to the oil. Soybeans and cruciferous vegetables such as broccoli and cabbage also contain lignans.

While lignan-rich foods are part of a healthful dietary pattern, it is possible to consume too many lignans. More than 45-50g per day of flaxseed may increase stool frequency or cause diarrhea in an adult. The safety of lignan supplements in pregnant or lactating women has not been established. Therefore, lignan supplements should be avoided by women who are pregnant, breast-feeding, or trying to conceive.

Phytates, also known as Phytic Acid, and Vitamin H—a form of inositol—may be considered a phytonutrient, providing an antioxidant and anti-inflammatory effect.

Researchers believe phytic acid, found in the fiber of legumes and grains, is the major ingredient responsible for preventing colon and other types of cancers. It may also help prevent cardiovascular disease and lower a food's glycemic load.

Phytates may have the ability to bind to certain dietary minerals including iron, zinc, manganese, and to a lesser extent calcium, and slow their absorption. However, the presence of phytates in foods really is not something to be concerned about as most people consume enough minerals in their diet to make up for any transitory deficiency. As long as a person eats a balanced diet, consuming too much phytates should not be a problem. The only folks who might need to be careful are vegetarians who consume a lot of wheat bran, which is a concentrated source of phytates.

Cooking reduces the phytic acid content in food to some degree, as does soaking whole grains prior for use in baking. To help this breakdown, you can soak them in yogurt, buttermilk, or water combined with lemon juice or vinegar.

Anthocyanidin-Rich Foods

Several fruits and vegetables contain high amounts of anthocyanidins. Some of the top anthocyanidin-rich foods are:

- *Blueberries carry a powerful blend of anthocyanidins and other antioxidants under their indigo skins.*
- *Red and black grapes make wine, in moderation, a potential health booster.*
- *Cranberries are so strongly flavored that they may need additional sugar or other complementary flavors.*
- *Raspberries and blackberries are a great source of antioxidants, especially when they are in season.*
- *Red cabbage is delicious when shredded in soups, salads or other dishes.*
- *Red onions are often served raw or with other vegetables and fruits.*
- *Eggplant can be roasted whole; the skin contains the antioxidants.*

Isothiocyanates (also known as mustard oils) impart characteristic flavors to such vegetable foods as wasabi, horseradish, mustard, radish, Brussels sprouts, watercress, nasturtiums, and capers. These various species generate different isothiocyanates in different proportions, and so have different, but recognizably related, flavors.

Some isothiocyanates may help prevent certain types of cancer by promoting the elimination of potential carcinogens from the body. However, they have a potentially goitrogenous effect on the thyroid. (Goitrogens are naturally-occurring substances that can interfere with function of the thyroid gland.) People with potential thyroid conditions should be careful when eating these foods.

Isothiocyanates appear to be sensitive to heat, so cooking cruciferous vegetables appears to lower the availability of isothiocyanates and their harmful effects. In the case of cruciferous vegetables like broccoli, as much as one third of this goitrogenic substance may be neutralized when broccoli is boiled in water.

In the absence of thyroid problems, there is no research evidence to suggest that goitrogenic foods will negatively impact health. In fact, the opposite is true: fermented soy foods and cruciferous vegetables have unique nutritional value, and the consumption of these foods has been associated with decreased risk of disease in many research studies.

There are varying opinions among healthcare professionals as to whether a person, who has thyroid problems, and notably a thyroid hormone deficiency, should limit their intake of goitrogenic foods. A wise course of action may be that people with thyroid problems should be cautious of an overconsumption of goitrogens. Here the goal is not to eliminate goitrogenic foods from the meal plan, but to cook them properly to limit intake so that it falls into a reasonable range.

Phenols are a large class of phytonutrients that exhibit a disease preventive character. Specifically, they have an outstanding ability to block certain enzymes that cause inflammation, therefore having

Studies have illustrated that saponins potentially have the ability to "clean" or purge these fatty compounds from the body.

the ability to protect human tissues from the damaging effects of oxidative stress. They can be found in berries, grapes, and purple eggplant, which receive their blue or blue-red color from their phenolic content. Bilberries also have a high phenolic character, their red color coming from the anthocyanidins they contain.

Many people use hydrogen peroxide for personal hygiene. Most external uses of household-strength hydrogen peroxide are relatively harmless. It can be useful as a gargle, an antiseptic for external wounds, an aid for removal of ear wax, bleach for hair and clothes, but do not drink it or inject it. Its internal use can be dangerous.

Saponins are "nature's detergents," having a soapy character. Because they have both water *and* fat soluble components, saponins are able to break down certain molecules, such as bile acids and cholesterols, lowering the blood lipids, cancer risks, and blood glucose levels more completely than either one could alone. They may also help fight inflammation and eczema, build bone health and stimulate the immune response.

Many vegetables are abundant in saponins, including beans, such as peas and soybeans, and herbs, like alfalfa and agave. Also, the saponins from the bulbs of red onions provide an antispasmodic effect. Certain saponins can also be found in herbs such as bacopa, fenugreek, ginseng, and tribulus. The herb Foxglove contains a saponin that benefits the heart—this is the fundamental source of the drug Digitalis®—which has been shown to strengthen and regulate contractions of the heart muscle, benefitting those with heart disease. Digitalis®-type saponins can be toxic in high doses and should only be used with professional supervision.

Several classes of saponins actually aid the absorption of important minerals, while others have anti-microbial

> *Glutathione is the most ubiquitous substance in the human system.*

properties particularly against fungi, bacteria, and certain parasites.

Other Phytonutrients

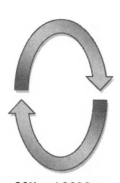

GSH and GSSG must be recycled in order for them to work together.

Glutathione—the reduced form, commonly abbreviated as GSH—is a unique molecule that plays a fundamental role in numerous metabolic and biochemical reactions. GSH is neither a vitamin nor an essential nutrient. It behaves more like a phytonutrient substance and is found everywhere in the body, helping many different systems work. While GSH is not a true protein, it contains an unusual molecular grouping of three commonly found amino acids (glutamic acid, glycine, and cysteine) joined by a special type of organic bond. GSH must be free to become oxidized—referred to as GSSG—to do its job of protecting the tissues, and then it must quickly revert back to its reduced state. If it becomes unstable or if the cofactors necessary to change GSH to GSSG and back again are not available, then it affects the ability of GSH to protect the tissues.

GSH is the major antioxidant produced *by the cells themselves*, protecting important cellular components against damage caused by free radicals. It eliminates many

> *Any antioxidant, cofactor or phytonutrient deficiency can allow free radicals to flourish.*

foreign compounds and carcinogens, both organic and inorganic. It helps protect cells from oxidative breakdown by poisons such as free radicals and peroxides (chemical compounds that contain oxygen atoms in the group—O_2—e.g., hydrogen peroxide, H_2O_2) that might attack from within one's own body. Every system in the human body is responsive to the state of GSH's presence, especially the immune system, the nervous system, the gastrointestinal system, and the lungs, but the largest reservoir of GSH is the liver. This is yet another reason to be sure tissue oxygen is metabolized properly, so that plenty of GSH persists.

> *Metabolic pathways must run their full course to maintain health. These pathways consume and produce energy, many times through oxidative means. Antioxidants help control those reactions, but too many antioxidants can quench the process with a harmful result. What was meant for good could produce harm when taken unwisely.*

The quantity of GSH in the tissues depends upon the availability of the many big-long-named cofactors necessary for its production. As the tissue levels of GSH rise to a given level, the mechanism eventually turns itself off; the blending of the amino acids is self-limiting. Fasting, protein-energy malnutrition (PEM), or other dietary amino acid deficiencies tend to limit GSH production. While the homeostatic GSH mechanisms always strive to be sure there is enough GSH available to the tissues, any direct attack by free radicals and other oxidative agents eventually deplete GSH. That stresses the production mechanisms to generate more GSH from foods, but these production pathways are limited and any prolonged oxidative depletion can outpace synthesis.

GSH is essential to cellular (or humeral, i.e., body fluids, especially blood serum) immunity. It helps some of the most powerful white blood cells linger when and where needed, and regulates the elimination of dead or damaged cells, and in this way maintains control of the immune response. If glutathione metabolism breaks down for any reason, the whole human system suffers. The point is that any antioxidant, cofactor or phytonutrient deficiency can allow free radicals to flourish.

Coenzyme Q10 (CoQ10) is an oil-soluble vitamin-like substance, present in the membranes of the many *organelles*—a smaller and specialized part of a cell that has a specific function—of most cells, primarily in the mito-

> Coenzyme Q10 is a natural vitamin-like antioxidant found in every cell of the body. It is thought to safeguard sharp thinking by protecting mitochondria, the power centers of the cells.

chondria. It acts inside the mitochondria along the electron transport chain during the production of ATP, and it participates in aerobic cellular respiration. Aerobic metabolism is responsible for about 95% of the human body's energy. Therefore, those organs with the highest energy requirements—such as the heart, the liver, and the brain—have the highest CoQ10 concentrations.

> It is a general rule in physiology: whatever you do to your brain you also do to your heart, and vice versa. Whether your brain changes relative to what you think, what you do, or what you eat, everything you consume eventually ends up in every cell and tissue of your body. So it makes sense to eat right for a healthy brain.

Recent clinical studies indicate that supplementation with CoQ10 may be of benefit to certain patients with congestive heart failure. Pending further medical studies, some medical groups have taken exception to some of these conclusions. However, many nutrition-minded doctors are beginning to recognize the possible benefits of CoQ10 in some heart and cardiovascular patients. Some doctors are also using CoQ10 to treat heart failure, migraine headaches, cardiac arrest, blood pressure, some cancers, and to enhance lifespan. However, much more research must be done before this sort of treatment becomes mainstream.

Eating plenty of fresh, raw, and unprocessed fish like sardines and mackerel; or meats like beef heart and liver; or fresh cuts of lamb and pork portions can help the body make CoQ10. Eggs provide the nutrients that help your body's mitochondria make your bodily systems run. Spinach and broccoli, wheat germ, fresh peanuts, and unprocessed whole grains give the body smaller ingredients that will enhance the probability that you are making and using CoQ10.

Medical literature has no long-term studies regarding toxicity from an overdose of alpha-lipoic acid, however, there have been no studies done with pregnant and lactating women so their use of alpha-lipoic acid supplements is not recommended.

It is worth knowing that cooking by frying reduces CoQ10 content by 15 to 30%. Further, there are many different factors affecting the concentration of CoQ10. The use of statin drugs, for example, reduces CoQ10 as does its exposure to ultraviolet light. And any person older than twenty years tends to have less CoQ10 in their organs, so it is generally good to be sure that you get plenty of CoQ10 after your second decade.

Lipoic Acid (also known as alpha-lipoic acid) is a fatty acid naturally occurring inside every cell in the body. It is essential to life and every aerobic process in order to produce the energy for normal cellular respiration. Lipoic acid helps convert glucose (blood sugar) into energy via aerobic means.

The antioxidant properties of lipoic acid help control the potentially harmful effects of free radicals. Unlike the well-known antioxidants such as Vitamins A, B, C, and E, lipoic acid functions in both water and fat. It also appears to be able to recycle antioxidants such as Vitamin C and glutathione after they have been utilized by the body.

The human system appears to be able to make lipoic acid on its own. It can also be found in very small amounts in spinach, broccoli, peas, Brewer's yeast, Brussels sprouts, rice bran, and organ meats. Many people add lipoic acid to their diet with supplements.

Although there is little doubt that antioxidants are a necessary component for good health, no one knows if supplemental antioxidants should be taken and, if so, how much. Antioxidant supplements were once thought to be harmless, but clinicians are becoming increasingly aware of interactions and potential toxicity.

It is interesting to note that in the normal concentrations found in the body, Vitamin C and beta-carotene are antioxidants; but at higher concentrations they are pro-oxidants and, thus, potentially harmful. Also, very little is known about the

> *Antioxidants are responsible for limiting the gusto of oxidative reactions, but megadoses of antioxidants can quench these very important reactions.*

long term consequences of megadoses of antioxidants. The body's finely tuned mechanisms are carefully balanced to withstand a variety of insults. Taking chemicals without a complete understanding of all of their effects may disrupt this balance.

This short list of phytonutrients is by no means complete. There are literally thousands of these living nutrients, each having its own specific protective effect on human tissues. Sadly, manufracturing renders the great majority of them useless, so it is of the utmost importance to be sure to eat right and know what you are eating.

Water: The Universal Solvent

> *Liquid water flows, but the quality of the water depends upon its viscosity, i.e., resistance to flow. The wetter the water the easier it flows; its molecules are rather loosely joined together. The sensation of wetness is largely due to the cooling caused by evaporation.*

The brain demands the most nourishment of any other tissue in the human body, and water is a very high priority. In total, there are about 70 trillion cells in the adult human body, made up of 30% mass—both protein and muscle—and the other 70% is water.

Most of all the water in the human system is salt water, not just water. It is a mineral-rich environment that is much different than pure water. Therefore, it may seem elementary, but water is an essential component for human physiology. And it makes sense that the *quality* of water should be equally as important as its *quantity*.

In general, water that is fit to drink—potable water—can be used with low risk of im-

> *Water exposed to air becomes more acidic from its exposure to carbon dioxide.*

mediate or long term harm, but most health-conscious people want more from their water. They want to ensure that the most valuable substance in their body will sustain proper health and wellness. To be sure, the water we drink should always be clean and free from contaminants.

Cellular transport systems, protection, and metabolism all depend upon a clean source of water. Clean water is as important for healthy tissues as are proper food, hygiene, and the avoidance of risky foods.

The Quality of Water

Many nutrients contribute to healthy brain function, each of them providing their essential components for repair that can optimize human performance. A

> *Obesity decreases the percentage of water in the body, sometimes to as low as 45%.*

healthy brain requires adequate amounts of available oxygen, vitamin complexes, essential fatty acids, amino acids (which will be discussed in the next chapter), micronutrients, minerals, and water. Nutritional experts agree that the brain requires proper nourishment for its continued health and youthfulness.

> *To estimate how many ounces of water a 200 pound man should consume in a day, divide the body weight by two; about 100 ounces of water in a day—about three quarts or three liters.*

One important problem affecting the quality of our water supply is the recent findings of trace elements of dozens of drugs in municipal water systems. Prescription drugs for every kind of malady make their way into the sink faucet: from neuroleptics to antibiotics to hormones and cancer drugs. The problem is becoming so significant that the federal government has finally convened a task force to study the risks posed by pharmaceuticals in the environment. Yet five years after it began its work, a new report by the Government Accountability Office is no closer to deciding whether these poisons should be regulated by the Clean Water Act.

There appears to be no standard for how much of these pharmaceutical pollutants are acceptable in the nation's rivers and streams or in the water that comes out of Americans' taps. Presumably, the extent of the pollution and whether it is a public health danger remains unclear, and these government agencies have never released their draft report due in part to internal squabbling.

The total amount of water in a man of average weight (150 pounds, or 70 kilograms) is approximately 40 liters—just over 10.5 gallons—averaging 57% of his total body weight. A newborn infant's percent water to body weight may be as high as 75%, but it gradually decreases from birth to old age, most of the decrease occurring during the first ten years of life.

The Quantity of Water

An abundant supply of good, clean water is crucial for good health, yet the average person's needs vary from day to day. Your daily water needs depend on many factors, including how healthy and how active you are, and the type of climate in which you live.

We have learned the importance of phytofoods, phytonutrients, phytochemicals, and "superfoods," and while not a micronutrient by any means, water is an essential aid in helping the brain "catch its breath"; it is vital for memory. Water makes up most of the blood components,

The nature of rock is to be hard, of grass to be green. The nature of water is to be wet. To take away from water's true nature is to destroy what it is and thus, it is no longer water.

and water's quantity is regulated by hormones, including the naturally occurring anti-diuretic hormone (ADH), as well as aldosterone and atrial natriuretic peptide (ANP). The brain and spinal cord require a large volume of water inside and surrounding it not only for the transport of various compounds, but also for protection. If your brain could speak, it would probably say, "I want to get wet!" A dehydrated brain releases the hormone cortisol, which negatively affects the brain's capacity to store information and create memory; too much cortisol tends to perpetuate stress.

Blood is comprised mainly of water, carrying oxygen, energy, and nutrients throughout the body. Water also plays a key role in cell metabolism, moving materials into and out of the cell. You can help your tissues regain the balance nature intended by drinking water; just plain water, with nothing else added.

In order for water to do its job it must be "wet" enough to penetrate to the deepest levels of tissue. That requires a very low viscosity— i.e., water has to be free-flowing. However, when water's surface tension becomes too high, it cannot infiltrate the tissues properly, causing a functional dehydration at deeper cellular levels. Only low viscosity water can regenerate even the deepest thirsty cells and make possible the elimination of toxic wastes from the cellular depths.

To function properly, the body requires between one and seven liters of water per day to avoid dehydration; the precise amount depends on the level of activity, the ambient and body temperature, the percentage of humidity, and several other factors. However, there appear to be no hard and fast rules regarding daily water consumption. The popular claim that "a person should consume eight glasses of water per day" seems to have no real basis in science.

> *It is not good for the brain to want water; thirst is very hard on the human brain.*

Similar misconceptions concerning the effect of water on weight loss and constipation have also been dispelled. However, it has been estimated that people should have an ounce of water for every kilogram (2.2 pounds) of their body weight per day. Most advocates agree that approximately two liters (eight-eight ounce glasses) of water daily is the minimum water consumption to maintain proper hydration. This is a good guideline and should be adjusted relative to your intake of other fluids, including ice cubes in non-water drinks. Most water is ingested through foods or beverages other than drinking straight water. Some medical literature, however, favors a lower consumption, typi-

> *"While city councils and water boards tend to fluoridate when they have the power, the electorate is far more divided. Over the past five years, the practice was voted down in 38 of 79 referendums, from Modesto, Calif., to Worcester, Mass."*
>
> —TIME Magazine, October 24, 2005

cally one liter of water for an average male, excluding extra requirements due to fluid loss from exercise or warm weather.

Even mild dehydration can drain your energy and make you feel tired. Typical symptoms of mild dehydration include headaches, sleepiness, and dizziness. Actual dehydration, or lack of water in the body, has a harmful impact on learning, so students should always drink more water.

For those who have healthy kidneys, it is rather difficult to drink too much water, but (especially in warm humid weather and while exercising) it is dangerous to drink too little. However, even people with normal kidneys can drink far more water than necessary while exercising, putting them at risk of water intoxication (hyperhydration), which can be fatal. There are several notable deaths from mineral depletion secondary to hyperhydration.

Water is lost during the course of a normal day through breathing, sweating, urination, and bowel movements, yet it does not cause constipation. Minerals such as sodium, potassium, and calcium (essential electrolytes) that maintain fluid balance in the body can also be lost. If too much water is lost and/or if the sensitive electrolyte balance is disturbed, the tissues become dehydrated. The young and the elderly are extremely susceptible to dehydration.

Fluoride in Your Water

> *The label on Crest®, America's favorite toothpaste reads:*
>
> *"Do not swallow."*
>
> *How about you? Do you swallow toothpaste? How about your kids? How can you be sure?*

One of the most toxic substances ever added to the public water supply is fluoride; i.e., sodium fluoride—the standard by which other water-fluoridation compounds are gauged. It is a known toxic chemical byproduct of the manufacturing of aluminum and phosphate fertilizer, cement, steel, and nuclear weapons; and it has been added to municipal water systems for the past fifty years. It made its way into the public water supply through big money and its influence on professional schools that are said to be responsible for the care of our teeth.

> *Of all the known minerals, fluoride has the greatest affinity to attract electrons toward itself; e.g., it can quickly attach itself to almost any other atom.*

However, since the early 1990s, literally hundreds of cities worldwide have taken a stand against further fluoridation of the public water system. Let the associations and municipalities say what they like, the fact remains that fluoride is a very toxic substance. In fact, the fluoridation issue is gaining so much momentum that it has been dubbed, *"Fluoridegate."*

Many public health experts believe that the addition of fluoride to drinking water helps prevent tooth decay and promotes overall dental health. Other equally expert health officials contend that fluoride not only does not prevent tooth decay, but it can contribute to other more serious health problems. It has been reported to cause brain damage, thyroid problems, and cancer.

In fact, many American Dental Association publications, for example, state that people with diabetes should drink "lots" of wa-

> *Some people believe that we should never put something in our mouth if we have to spit it out.*

ter, but fail to share that the water should be unfluoridated. "Lots" of fluoridated (tap) water means "lots" of fluoride, and fluoride is a cumulative poison that collects in bones, joints, and the pineal gland. Further, the Gerber® baby products company has started selling unfluoridated water (Gerber® Pure™ Water) so that parents of young babies will not use fluoridated water when mixing milk formula. Finally, since diabetes is characterized by an increased thirst, more water means more fluoride.

> *Almost any form of a substance may be absorbed through the mucous membranes underneath the tongue if it dissolves easily in saliva. Toothpastes and mouth washes are designed for solubility. As a result, because of the rich supply of capillaries underneath the tongue, sublingual absorption is much faster than through the stomach, i.e., toothpastes and mouth washes that contain fluoride can be absorbed quite easily through the mouth.*

Noting that various fluoride types can cause a permanent disfiguring staining of teeth called "dental fluorosis," a bipartisan group from the Tennessee House of Representatives has apparently written a letter to State Health Commissioner Susan Cooper, asking that the Commissioner direct State Health Department employees to halt activities that promote the practice of water fluoridation. They expressed concern that "many Tennessee families are unaware" about Gerber's® unfluoridated water, and that citizens may not be able to afford unfluoridated water for their babies' formula, nor have the funds to repair fluorosis stains on their children's teeth.

The Tennessee legislators' letter pointed out that the National Research Council Committee for Fluoridation (2006) acknowledges kidney patients, diabetics, seniors, and babies to be "susceptible subpopulations" that are particularly vulnerable to harm from ingested fluorides. Further, the chairman of that committee stated in a

> *Fluorosilicic acid—known by several different scientific names: fluosilicic acid, hydrofluorosilic acid, silicofluoride, silicofluoric acid. It is related to one of the most dangerous acids—hydrogen fluoride—and the production of phosphate fertilizers. The majority of the hexafluorosilicic acid is used for the production of aluminum.*

January 2008 *Scientific American* article, "…when we looked at the studies that have been done, we found that many of these questions are unsettled and we have much less information than we should, considering how long this [fluoridation] has been going on."

In a January 2009 letter to the Vice President of Clinical Affairs of the American Dental Association, Daniel G. Stockin, MPH, a career public health professional with a strong background in hazardous materials management and toxics assessment, of the Lillie Center Inc., a firm working to end the practice of fluoridation, stated, "Fluorides are the next 'asbestos'. In fact, discussions with attorneys and my experience in the asbestos and lead fields indicate to me that fluoride harm represents even larger legal and financial liability than asbestos or lead." Stockin went on to say that, "The house of cards that is water fluoridation is wobbling and about to collapse." Water districts appear to be taking another look at their fluoridation practices, wondering what business they have medicating people through water.

Fluoride interrupts the last step of the metabolism of glucose to pyruvic acid, sending the metabolic pathways along a different course. As you recall, the Krebs cycle produces 36 molecules of ATP per molecule of glucose, but this fluoride-interrupted alternative pathway only produces four to six molecules of ATP for the same molecule of glucose. I do not know about you, but I would much rather forego the fluoride and its diversion, and end up with five to nine times the energy per molecule of glucose.

New York City Councilman Peter Vallone Jr. asked his constituents, "Did you know that the government is putting toxic chemicals in our water, which come from the scrubbing systems of the fertilizer industry and are classified as 'hazardous wastes' (sodium fluorosilicate and fluorosilicic acid)? Are you concerned? You should be. Unfortunately, when these chemicals are called 'fluoride,' safety concerns go down the drain." Vallone recently introduced a bill that would eliminate the addition of fluoride to city water supplies, claiming it "amounts to forced medication by the government."

> *Fluoride (F) is known to affect mineralizing tissues, but its effects upon the developing brain had not been previously considered until about 20 years ago when scientists found that fluoride exposures caused severe behavioral changes in rats, directly related to the levels of fluoride in specific brain regions. They considered these findings important because plasma levels in rats appear to be similar to those reported in humans exposed to high levels of fluoride.*

In another fluoride-related matter, the U.S. Health and Human Services Department recommended lowering previously-sanctioned amounts of fluoride in drinking water. Right after that, in January, 2011, the Environmental Protection Agency proposed doing away with the use of a fluoride-containing pesticide used in food storage and processing facilities.

Fluosilicic acid, which is a classified hazardous waste, is the substance used in 90% of the water fluoridation programs in the United States. Toothpastes and mouth washes often contain sodium fluoride or sodium monofluorophosphate (MFP) to prevent cavities, but the label cautions against swallowing the paste. (Sodium fluoride is related to rat poison.) It says, "If you accidentally swallow more than used for brushing, seek professional help or contact a poison control center immediately." Do you know the prescribed amount? Television commercials teach us to use a generous "S" shaped blob on the full length of the toothbrush. Again, the label says, "To minimize swallowing use a pea-sized amount and supervise brushing until good habits are established." Do not let your toothpaste's minty freshness fool you. You could probably consume six to eight pea-sized doses for every full brush blob, which is six to eight times the recommended dose per brushing. And they want you to dose yourself with that much sodium fluoride twice daily. How much do you use on your toothbrush? How much fluoride are you consuming?

Fluoride-containing substances can reduce IQ, impair memory and learning; fluoride has been shown to poison kidney function. It causes bone disease and reduced thyroid activity, and is a proven cause of cancer.

Proper nutrition and diet are no longer a goal, but a necessity for living well today. Contaminated air, water, and soil quality, and unhealthy lifestyles—fast foods, ignoring food labels, and eating manufractured foods—are taking their toll on our bodies down to the deepest cellular level.

Much has been written about the type of water to drink. Some sources say tap water is healthy, but copious news articles would disagree because of the drugs, chemicals, fluoride, and other products found in tap water. Some articles say bottled water is best, but then you have to consider the issue of leaching plastics. Other proponents of healthy water say you should only consume your water from glass bottles, but then the issues are weight and safety of the glass. But this water issue is far too complicated for us to definitively deal with here. Suffice it to say that the quality of water you consume is very important, and the reader is encouraged to do their homework before settling on any one source. Know the truth about the water you drink and why that truth is real.

Summary

Your brain's breath is vital to your healthiness. More than that, it is crucial for life! You probably already know that your brain cannot persist for more than a few minutes before critical life support systems shut down, then death. Your breath is your source of oxygen that is fundamental to everything human. Oxygen, fuel, and the avenue for delivery—a free-flowing vascular system—are essential to make the energy that drives all your systems.

You would think that your brain knows how to use the oxygen it receives. You might think that existence means at least some oxygen is reaching your brain. While that may be true, the question becomes one of oxygen saturation—how much oxygen is available. Of the oxygen that reaches your brain, how much of it is usable for your activities of daily living? Is a person with a low oxygen perfusion as vital as another person who can figure out complex mathematics, play a complicated piano masterpiece, or an Olympic athlete? Certainly not. Is that first person less human? No. That first person is still human, but they have a reduced capacity to express that humanity relative to another person who is more vital. Vitality is the difference. We are all human beings trying to reach our optimal potential, but that cannot happen when the ability to use oxygen is compromised.

Our available fuel comes from the items we consume. Foods—including herbs—provide vital phytonutrients essential for building and repairing all cells, and they make up all tissues. Water is essential for life, too. The quality and quantity of water you consume is directly related to your level of hydration. Water helps carry nutrients to their innermost destination and serves to wash toxins away from your cells and tissues.

Together, oxygen, water, and the delivery system to make it all happen are essential components for life. This is how your body produces the energy necessary to express your humanity. Your best source of energy comes from nutrient dense foods, and in the next chapter we will discuss your best energy source: fatty acids.

Interesting Brain Facts

- *The weight of the human brain averages about three pounds (1300-1400 grams)*
- *The relative weight of the neocortex at birth is about 12 ounces (350 grams), 25% of its adult weight*
- *The developing brain increases by 250,000 new cells every minute*
- *The weight of the cortex at 6 months is 50% of its adult weight**
- *The weight of the cortex at 30 months is about 75% of its adult weight*
- *At age 5 years (before school), the cerebral cortex is about 90% of its adult weight*
- *The brain represents about 2% of the total body weight independent of mental activity level, continuing even during sleep*
- *The adult human brain contains about 100 billion neurons*
- *Each neuron connects to between 1,000 and 10,000 other neurons*
- *The brain consumes about 25% of the total breathed oxygen*
- *The brain burns about 70% of all the available glucose in the body*
- *The brain uses about 25% of all the available nutrients in the body*
- *About 1.5 pints of blood traverse the cerebrum every minute*
- *There are about 100,000 miles of blood vessels, capillaries and other transport systems in the adult human brain*
- *If laid end to end, all the neurons of the human system would stretch 112,000 miles, enough to circle the globe five times at the equator*
- *There are about 1 quadrillion (one million billion) connections in the adult human brain*
- *The adult human cerebral cortex takes up 25% of the entire brain volume*
- *The adult human cerebral cortex houses about 80-85% of all the neurons in the brain*
- *The adult human cerebral cortex is about 1.5 to 4.5mm, or 1/8 inch in thickness (about the thickness of a dime)*
- *The adult human cerebral cortex has six different layers*

During the first 6 months of life, there is a massive increase in the weight of the developing young brain due to the myelination of the axons, along with the tremendous increase in the number of dendrites and glial cells. These events combine to generate a 1-milligram per minute growth rate in the young brain.

CHAPTER FOUR

FATTY ACIDS

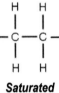

Saturated
Fatty Acid

Fatty acids (fats) are the building blocks of the fat in our bodies and they can come from either animal or vegetable sources. The term "fatty acids" relates to the way certain long chains of carbon molecules hook together, having certain biochemical traits. One such trait is the freedom of movement around single-bonded carbon atoms while double-bonded carbons resist this movement.

When fatty acids are found by themselves they are known as "free" fatty acids and they are important sources of fuel that yield large quantities of ATP. While carbohydrates are digested quickly, fats are the slowest to be broken down and absorbed. That means that carbohydrates provide quick energy while fatty acids yield energy more slowly.

These fatty acids provide the building blocks for cell membranes and an array of hormones, and they include the fat-soluble Vitamins A, D, E, and K.

In general terms, a fatty acid is a long unbranched chain of carbon atoms that can have single or double bonds between them, making them either saturated or unsaturated fats. A straight chain of single-bonded carbon atoms makes up a saturated fat. The chain that has double bonds is termed an unsaturated fat, and an unsaturated fat with two or more double bonds is polyunsaturated.

"Cis" versus "Trans" Fats

The differences in configuration between the *cis* and *trans* forms of unsaturated fatty acids, as well as between saturated and unsaturated fatty acids, play an important role in biological processes and in the construction of biological structures, such as a cellular membrane. Those configurations are important. The parts of a cell membrane should fit together like a jigsaw puzzle. When the essential molecule for membrane construction is available, the puzzle goes together like it should, but one misshapen part kinks up the whole works.

The Whole Configuration of a Saturated Fatty Acid

Most naturally-occurring unsaturated fatty acids have *cis* bonds—these are the good guys. In contrast, most fatty acids in the *trans* configuration—trans-fats—are *not* found in nature and are produced by man (e.g., hydrogenation; hydrogen atoms have filled all the available bonding slots).

"*Cis*" Configuration

The two ends of an unsaturated fatty acid—a fatty acid molecule that still has some available bonding slots—are not free to rotate around those unfilled slots like they can on a saturated fatty acid; a double bond holds the molecular configuration tightly. Those unfilled slots (*double bonds*) give unsaturated fatty acids a uniquely stable character. The rigidity of the double bond freezes the fatty acid's molecular arrangement. A *cis* configuration gives the fatty acid molecule a characteristic bend. The more double bonds along the *cis* chain, the more bends it has and the less flexible it is. This is important when it comes to the structural makeup of the cellular membrane.

"*Trans*" Configuration

The upshot is that, since *cis* bonds make the molecule more curved, these curves provide for openings in a cell's membrane. Their curved structure al-

> *A good health rule: If a nutrient is good for the heart, it is also good for the brain, and vice versa.*

lows more space between the fatty acids, which is important when you consider that fatty acids are a key component of the cell membrane. These spaces provide avenues to transport substances into, and wastes out of, the cells.

Conversely, a *trans* configuration puts the adjacent hydrogen atoms on the *opposite* of the double bond. There is no bend in the carbon chain, and their chain is much like that of straight saturated fatty acids. If the cell's membrane has no openings—because the diet did not provide the essential components to build the cells according to their original design—there cannot be intake of nutrients or the elimination of toxins. This is damaging to the cell.

Essential Fatty Acids

Almost all the polyunsaturated fats in the human diet are essential (EFAs), and they have an important part in many metabolic processes. Fatty acids are generally used as the source of fuel for the Krebs cycle, but the *essential* fatty acids are different because they are more often involved in biological processes, including vital brain functions and the life and death of heart cells.

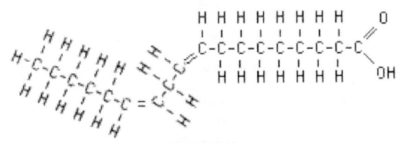

Linoleic Acid

Essential fatty acids—those fatty acids that cannot be made by the body—were first known as Vitamin F. Yes, Vitamin F is actually a vitamin! Since the EFA's discovery in 1923, their classification has changed, and they have been broken down into omega-3 and omega-6 fatty acids, each class being essential.

The main unsaturated fatty acids—oleic acid (OA), linoleic acid (LA), and alpha-linolenic acid (ALA)—have relatively short chains. Our bodies

The term "omega" when used relating to fatty acids, indicates the placement of the double bond, i.e., omega-3's have their double bond in the third position.

can make oleic acid, but it is thought that we are unable to create linoleic or alpha-linolenic acids—and that makes these latter two fatty acids essential.

Omega-3

Alpha-Linolenic Acid

Hooking two shorter chain unsaturated fatty acids together makes their chains longer, increasing their number of unsaturated bonds and making them polyunsaturated fatty acids (PUFAs). However, this conversion does not happen very easily. If the diet is missing any of these EFAs, their deficiency will eventually make its way to the cells, altering their structure and impeding their function. The nervous system can eventually show signs of learning disabilities and depression.

If your brain could speak it might say, "Take me to the beach," because seafoods and the oils they contain are very nourishing to the brain. The depression rate has been found to decrease as much as 60% as the consumption of fish increases. Omega-3 fatty acids are an essential component of the neurotransmitter serotonin, which is known to improve mood.

The three main desaturated omega-3 fatty acids are eicosapentaenoic acid (EPA), docosahexaenoic acid (DHA), and alpha-linolenic acid (ALA); but not

For the record, oleic acid has a "kink" with one double bond. Linoleic acid, with two double bonds, has a more pronounced curve, and alpha-linolenic acid, with three double bonds, favors a hooked shape.

EPA and DHA Oils

Oil from cold-water fish is a good source of both eicosapentaenoic (ei·co·sa·pen·ta·e·no·ic) acid (EPA) and docosahexaenoic (do·co·sa·hex·a·e·no·ic) acid (DHA). These oils come from cod, salmon, mackerel, herring, sardines, sablefish (black cod), anchovies, albacore tuna, and wild game.

EPA and DHA are vital nutrients to maintain healthy brain and heart function. They become hormone-like substances called prostaglandins, and they regulate cell activity and healthy cardiovascular function.

DHA is a building block of the brain and of the retina. It helps produce neurotransmitters, like phosphatidylserine, which is important for brain function. DHA is found in the retina of the eyes, and supplementing with DHA may be necessary for maintaining healthy levels of DHA for normal eye function.

Adding DHA to a pregnant mother's diet may be beneficial for the development of the fetus's brain. It plays a very important role during fetal development, early infancy, and old age. High concentrations of DHA are found in the brain, and DHA increases 300-500% in an infant's brain during the last trimester of pregnancy. Because our bodies make less EPA and DHA as we age, it may reduce mental focus and cognitive function. Taking EPA and DHA may also help with mental abnormalities, such as Alzheimer's disease and dementia.

EPA and DHA are a source of energy; they insulate the body against heat loss, prevent skin from drying and flaking, and cushion tissues and organs.

---

all omega-3s are the same. EPA and DHA are considered long-chain forms of omega-3 fats and are the most studied sources for health benefits. They are found in fish and fish oil supplements such as salmon, tuna, swordfish, anchovies, sardines, trout, herring, and algae extract; EPA is found in human breast milk, and DHA is a major fatty acid in sperm and brain phospholipids, and in the retina.

> It is thought that omega-3 fatty acids can help reduce arthritic inflammation—the inflammation of the joint between two bones. Omega-3 supplements can ease tenderness in joints, decrease stiffness, and reduce the need for anti-inflammatory medication.

DHA is an essential component of the human brain. Sixty percent of the brain is comprised of these omega-3 fatty acids. If insufficient amounts of these EFAs are consumed in the diet, the myelin sheath surrounding nerve and brain cells may be inadequate because there is not enough fat-rich myelin to complete the job according to the nerve's original design. Studies have shown that children with certain learning disabilities, such as attention deficit disorder (ADD), may be aided by ensuring that their diets are sufficient in omega-3 fatty acids.

Krill oil—fatty acids that come from a small shrimp-like zooplankton—may be one of the best sources of omega-3 fatty acids because krill has a lower metal content. Heavy metals such as lead, aluminum, chromium, mercury, etc. are harmful to humans.

Many researchers say that the American diet is deficient in ALA, which is involved with cell oxidation and metabolizing important sulphur-containing amino acids. It also plays a role in the production of special hormone-like molecules (prostaglandins) that are involved with controlling smooth muscle contraction, blood pressure, asthma, learning deficiencies, and heart disease.

ALA, the short-chain omega-3 fatty acid, is found in plant sources like walnuts, flax seed, chia seeds, citrus fruits, melons, cherries, canola, and soybean oil, and to a lesser degree in green leafy vegetables (like let-

> If you choose tuna (Albacore), and even if you buy the same brand of tuna all the time, the fat content can vary as much as two grams per ounce, depending upon the season the fish is caught, and water temperature. Further, be sure the tuna you buy is packed in water rather than oil. Water helps maintain the quality of omega-3s. Also, be sure to read the "Nutrition Facts" label on the products you buy because the data must tell you what nutrients have been added to the packaging.

tuce, broccoli, kale, purslane, and spinach), and legumes (like kidney, navy, pinto, and lima beans). While the body may be able to convert ALA into DHA and EPA, the process is very inefficient, and health experts generally recommend that foods rich in both DHA and EPA be obtained directly from their original food source at least two times a week.

While one omega-3 fatty acid can change to another omega-3 fatty acid, it is not possible to create omega-3 fatty acids from a fatty acid or from saturated fats. That makes the consumption of omega-3 fatty acids especially important.

Omega-6

The omega-6 fatty acid Linoleic Acid (LA) is an essential fatty acid; the body cannot create it. LA comes from most vegetable oils, like sunflower, safflower, corn, sesame oils, and black currant seeds. It can also be found in poultry, eggs from chickens kept in cages (perhaps because they obtain a different diet and exercise than cage-free chickens), whole-grain cereals and breads, pumpkin seeds, and nuts.

The desaturated—polyunsaturated—omega-6 fatty acids are GLA (gamma-linolenic acid), DGLA (dihomo-gamma-linolenic acid), and AA (arachidonic acid). The average diet provides plenty of omega-6 fatty acids, yet research says they are not necessarily good for your long-term health because they have a unique makeup that can lead to the production of pro-inflammatory factors.

The omega-6 fatty acids are found in vegetable oils, such as corn, soy, palm, sunflower, safflower, and rapeseed. Many refined vegetable oils, such as soybean oil, are used in most of the fast foods, snack foods, cookies, crackers, and sweets in the American diet. It is almost impossible to get away from dietary soybean oil. Omega-6 fatty acids account for an estimated 20% of the calories in the American diet. Can you imagine that?

Since omega-6 fatty acids are so readily available, it is generally recognized that they should be avoided if a person wants to stay healthy; because not all omega-6 fatty acids are good. Cardiovascular experts say that, at the most, the ratio of omega-6 and omega-3 fatty acids should be somewhere between 1:1 to 1:4. That means that these omega oils should be anywhere from equal ratios to one part omega-6 to four parts omega-3, and these levels can be tough to maintain unless you are paying close attention to everything you consume.

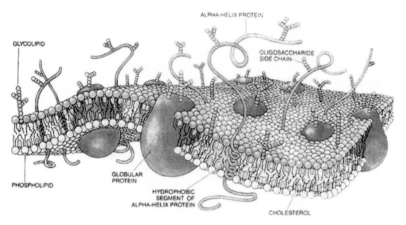

Complex cell membrane showing phospholipid membrane (credit: NIST)

The Cell Membrane Is Like A Double-Layered Sandwich
Each neuron has a thin, double-layered outer membrane that defines the nerve's borders. The outer membrane controls the flow of other substances (such as vitamins, minerals, proteins, etc.) into and out of the cell. The membrane is made of sandwiched layers of special fats (lipids, or fatty acids) and amino acids. Both come from the diet because the human system cannot make them. If they are not ingested, the membrane's integrity develops a lesser quality, and that eventually leads to disease.

Eating a diet high in omega-6 fats means that there is a greater possibility that those harmful fats will reach the cell membrane. That is where a delicate balance exists between omega-6 and omega-3 fatty acids, which affect nearly every biological function in one way or another. They check

> *Eating a diet high in omega-6 fats means that there is a greater possibility that those harmful fats will reach the cell membrane.*

each other as they regulate thousands of metabolic functions—like controlling smooth muscle contraction, blood pressure, inflammation, and body temperature. In general, both omegas work in a way similar to hormones to influence inflammation, modify mood and behavior, clarify cellular signaling, and modulate DNA activities. However, while both the omega-3 and omega-6 fatty acids help reduce inflammation, under certain conditions the omega-6 fatty acids have a character that can also *lead* to inflammation. Too much omega-6 fats can interfere with the health benefits of omega-3 fats, partly because they compete for the same enzymes. A shift toward omega-6 fats in the diet tends to create a physiological state that favors diseases that lead to thrombosis, inflammation, and constriction.

A Balancing Act

Most commercial vegetable oils have very little omega-3 ALA and way too much omega-6 LA. Further, modern food production practices have processed much of the omega-3 fatty acids out of commercially available vegetables, eggs, fish, and

> *Where the omega-3 and omega-6 fats are balanced, the cell can work relatively efficiently. However, any imbalance here makes the cell membrane less able to protect the interior of the cell from invasion by unwanted materials and/or eliminate toxic products.*

meat. Free-range chicken eggs, from hens that eat a more natural diet of insects and green plants, seem to contain higher levels of omega-3 oils than eggs from caged chickens. Free-range eggs are apparently richer in omega-3 oils so their consumption must be monitored. Commercial supermarket eggs can contain as much as nineteen times more omega-6 than omega-3. Milk and cheese from grass-fed cows may also be a good source of omega-3 fatty acids; pasteurization can negatively affect their nutrient's quality.

Overall low levels of EFAs—or the wrong balance of omega-3 to omega-6 fatty acids—may have extremely toxic health effects. Omega-3 fatty acids can be found in the most metabolically active cells of a living organism. Omega-3 fats appear to speed up the activity of cells. When diets are deficient in omega-3 fatty acids, it is correlated with a lowered metabolism, which can lead to weight gain. It is quite possible that over 90% of the adults in the United States consume too few omega-3 fatty acids, contributing to heart attacks, thrombotic stroke, arrhythmia, arthritis, osteoporosis, inflammation, mood disorders, obesity, and even some cancers.

> In the United States, oil labeling is not regulated, so "cold pressed oil" may not actually be cold pressed oil at all. Consumers will need to smell, taste, and see the oil to determine whether or not it is truly cold pressed.

Where the omega-3 and omega-6 fats are balanced, the cell can work relatively efficiently. However, any imbalance here makes the cell membrane less able to protect the interior of the cell from invasion by unwanted materials and/or eliminate toxic products. Elevated tissue omega-6 levels can increase the tendency to clot formation, high blood pressure, inflammation, digestive tract irritation, immune depression, sterility, cell proliferation, cancer, and weight gain.

Consuming the oil of a product is not the same thing as eating the raw or roasted seeds or nuts. Human teeth cannot chew the food fine enough to break open the cells that contain the oils. Further, roasting seeds and nuts degrades the flavor, nutritional value, and color of the oil, altering the configuration of the food's oils making them less nutritious than they are in their raw form. Therefore, the best way to obtain these seed and nut oils is after they have been cold or expeller pressed, generally below normal body temperature depending on the oil, but is generally around 80° F (27° C).

It may seem contradictory, except for those reasons above, omega-6 fats *do* have a place in a healthy diet; their consumption needs to be monitored. In general, eat more cold-water fish, nuts and seeds, fresh fruits and vegetables, proteins, whole grains, and take essential fatty acid supplements. Your brain also appreciates fewer saturated fats (meat and dairy products).

Omega-9

Fatty acids can also be classified as omega-9 (monounsaturated oleic acid), which dramatically reduce the body's inflammatory response.

Omega-9 EFAs are generally available in the balanced human diet. It can be found in extra virgin olive oil, olives, avocados, almonds, peanuts, sesame oil, pecans, pistachio nuts, cashews, hazelnuts, macadamia nuts, etc.

Any oil you buy should be organic and expeller-pressed. Lesser quality products sold in supermarkets have a high probability of having been extracted with chemical solvents or high-speed presses that generate heat. Both the chemical and high-speed press methods alter the oil's fatty acid chemistry in undesirable ways, which can lead to adverse side effects.

One to two tablespoons of extra virgin or virgin olive oil per day should provide plenty oleic acid for adults. However, the "time-released" effects of obtaining these nutrients from nuts and other whole foods is thought to be more beneficial than consuming the entire daily amount through a single dose of oil.

There is evidence that humans are generally able to make omega-9s, provided there are ample essential fatty acids in their diet. Some exceptions might occur in older people or people with liver problems. Therefore, many supplement companies produce and sell omega 3-6-9 blends.

Making Cold Pressed Oils

Know your oil terms: "cold pressed oil" is subject to different regulations, depending on where it is made. "Expeller pressed oil" is created in a high pressure environment, and pressure creates heat that can make the oil rancid. Some expeller pressed oil can be termed cold pressed, but not if it reaches high temperatures. To be candid about their quality, some companies make their processing techniques very clear by specifically labeling their product, "expeller cold pressed oil."

The nuts, seeds, or fruits used to make oil are first ground into an even paste. The paste goes through a kneading, rubbing or massaging process; it is much like a slow stirring that encourages the oil in the paste to clump. Pressure is applied to the mixture, forcing the oil out of the paste. However, this process is delicate because pressure and force create friction and heat. While heating the paste may increase the yield of oil, heat can also damage the oil's quality. Some producers mix the paste with warm water, or heat it before pressing. Others make cold pressed oil by using a stone with a fine grain lubricated with oil alone to remove the desired oil. After the sought oil has been produced, it is graded and bottled.

Canola Oil

Canola oil is a contrived substance unfit for human consumption. Here's why: In the 1980s, polyunsaturated fats were all the rage, but they were not delivering the hyped health benefits. However, since food scientists had made such a big deal about the dangers of saturated fats, they could not reverse their

> *All nuts, and walnuts (which are actually seeds), "feed your brain" because they keep your arteries clear and boost serotonin levels. Serotonin is a neurotransmitter that controls sleep, depression, memory, and other neurological processes. Raw unprocessed organic olive oil, coconut oil and hempseed oil also contain brain healthy fats, fibers, and proteins.*

course and admit their error. Instead, they began to stimulate and educate the consumer about the health benefits of canola oil while at the same time magnifying the deadly hazards of saturated fats. The authorities said saturated fats would kill us. The message became increasingly distorted by the food processing industry with the discovery that canola oil's characteristics were much like those of margarine—and that alone could make the food industry more money and extend the shelf life of supermarket items. However, prolonging shelf life only means that food has minimal liveliness, if any at all.

Canola's Characteristics

Canola oil is the trade name for the oil made from rapeseed, which naturally contains erucic acid, a fatty acid, and is poisonous to humans because of its association with fibrous legions of the heart, Vitamin E deficiency, undesirable changes in the blood platelets and shortened life-span.

Rapeseed—which is related to turnip, rutabaga, cabbage, kale, Brussels sprouts, mustard greens, and many other vegetables—has been

> *Canola Oil® is an excellent example of a previously toxic substance being brought to the human food chain through genetic manipulation. Food scientists have probably exchanged rapeseed oil's poisonous erucic acid content for a more subtle and dangerous type of toxicity.*

routinely used in Asian cooking for generations, perhaps because it was consumed in low quantities immediately after crushing by hand and at very low temperatures. They certainly did not deep fry with it, genetically engineer it, use solvents to extract it potentially leaving behind toxic hexane solvents used for its extraction, deodorize it—which renders most of its omega-3s rancid—and hydrogenate it. However, the newer manufacturing techniques—genetic modification—that virtually eliminate the toxic erucic acid content (LEAR: Low Erucic Acid Rapeseed) have changed canola's natural molecular structure into a fabricated substance with a character different than its original design. Before it could be brought to the marketplace, the LEAR oil had to be renamed, hence: Canadian oil of low acid, Canola® oil.

This once poisonous LEAR substance has become Generally Recognized as Safe (GRAS) by the USDA since about 1985. The process used to genetically modify the rapeseed apparently lowers the erucic acid content from 45% to less than 25% as found in common cano-

> *Some canola oil products have been chemically manipulated by refinement and processing to withstand temperatures of up to 520°F. Therefore, although there is a 2:1 ratio of omega-6 to omega-3 fatty acids, canola oil must be used cold or it is of little use, and its levels of trans-fats exceeds that of margarine.*

la oil. Further, this new rapeseed was bred to have a fatty acid profile of just over 50% monounsaturated fat.

Canola oil is a rich source of omega-6 polyunsaturated fatty acids—24% omega-6 fatty acids and 10% omega-3 fatty acids; just over a 2:1 ratio. However, studies show that excessive consumption of these omega-6 fatty acids can be counterproductive since they can produce inflammation. Further, it is canola oil's omega-3 content that makes it unsafe to heat, producing a hydrogenated and dangerous *trans* form of fat, rancid and foul smelling when heated above 120°F. This hydrogenation extends canola's shelf life, making it a very attractive food additive.

Consumer Caution Advised

> It is also quite probable that canola products have high levels of pesticides used by canola oil producers, opening the way for possible tainting of the finished product. Be sure to check the product's label carefully.

Consumers should be very cautious about using canola oil. Today, canola oil is found in almost every food on store shelves—even health food stores. Despite its lowered erucic acid content, the widespread inclusion of canola oil into most every manufactured grocery item may lead to heart damage and liver trouble. Recall the similar argument made with the injudicious fluoridation of water. The idea may be good; the application is twisted with danger. Although some researchers have contested these findings, other authorities believe that the consumption of smaller amounts of erucic acid is harmless.

The regular use of canola oil can cause a wide array of side effects. Various problems arise because no two people are ever alike. Some people's livers, for example, may be able to clear the toxic effects of rapeseed relatively well

> Stay healthy by heating and/or cooking with organic, extra virgin cold pressed unrefined coconut oil. Use organic olive oil on your salads, but do not heat it. Use coconut oil for everything. It is very tasty with a slight hint of coconut. Throw away any oil that smokes; it is toxic.

while other people may have a greater sensitivity to it resulting in liver congestion. These supposedly harmless toxins (i.e., erucic acid) still have to be broken down and metabolized by the liver and other eliminative organs, despite their lowered presence. Even the most balanced metabolic pathways eventually become symptomatic as toxicity eats away at the fabric of wellbeing; the systems eventually falter. When the essential components for repair are unavailable, it leads to breakdown of the detoxification pathways discussed by Beardall, with eventual sickness and disease.

A Little History Lesson

Historically, canola plants were originally hybridized to modify their quality, but the genetic modification of canola, which increases their resistance to herbi-

There are few studies to evaluate the effects of erucic acid on humans, the majority being done by the food science industry on animals.

cide, was first introduced to Canada in the mid 1990's. Today, 80% of the canola acres sown are genetically engineered. This genetically engineered end result is not like that which was originally hybridized by grafting.

Generally, both hybridization and genetic engineering produce the same end result—new genetic types. The difference, however, is in the process.

Hybrid (or recombinant) plants come from seeds that are the product of cross-pollination of specific parental types—the hybrid gets half of its genes from each parent—so that the resulting crops will have certain genetic vitality. While there may be some artificial insertion of genetic material into today's hybrids, generally speaking, they are not genetically engineered, that is, the process does not use high-tech or biotechnology.

The food industry tries to make us believe ingredients like canola oil, Aspartame® or NutraSweet®, soybean oil, Olestra®, and Splenda® are healthy for you but, in actuality, they are not. They can actually be quite dangerous to our biological systems.

On the other hand, genetic engineering usually refers to the biotechnology used to manipulate the genetic encoding material (DNA) of one plant with the genetic framework of another plant related to a biological feature desired in the original plant. This whole new plant is unlike any made by nature—a genetically modified organism, or GMO. The two plants are nearly identical, except for the gene or genes that were technologically inserted.

Despite all the efforts to keep the two types of canola apart—hybridized and GMO—there are cases of cross-contamination of regular canola oil crops from the nearby genetically modified fields, which appears to have been a serious problem for Canadian canola farmers. It can be very difficult for farmers to grow hybridized crops, or non-genetically modified (non-GMO) crops because of the frequent contamination by the wind-blown pollens from the genetically modified fields. To date, no courts have resolved the issue and the problem continues.

As I See It

This concerns me: How can a product claim to be called "organic" if its origins are founded through genetic manipulation?

Unprocessed canola oil, which cannot be found in our natural food supply, does contain high levels of both monounsaturated fats and omega-3 fatty acids, but not so with the processed variety, the most common one. My recommendation is to stay completely away from canola oil. Heart controversies aside, the human liver has trouble metabolizing canola oil, and that can lead to other subtler—and more serious—reactions in the end.

Summary

Healthy fatty acids provide the essential components for needed energy and to repair and rebuild resilient cell membranes. However, not just any fats will suffice. In general, you are wise to consume the *cis* form of fatty acids and avoid the *trans* form. The *cis* fatty acids conform to the original design of vital tissues to increase resistance against the damaging effects of wear and tear while the *trans* form eventually leads to adaptation and breakdown. *Trans* fats become lodged in the fabric of the cell membrane making it less flexible and increasing the tendency to cellular toxicity.

Further, be sure to maintain the appropriate ratio between omega-3 and omega-6 fats. The former are more suitable because they can better accommodate pain control while the latter can contribute to degenerative conditions leading to adaptation. According to most cardiologists, the healthiest ratio of omega-3 to omega-6 approaches three or four to one. This is where each can provide its greatest benefit with the least negative effects.

The general rule here is to know what types of fats you are consuming. Enjoy the healthy fats and avoid the unhealthy ones. Most importantly, avoid canola oil. It is a man-made concoction, having no place in a healthy person's diet.

CHAPTER FIVE

HEART HEALTH IS BRAIN-BASED

Preventing Heart Attacks: A New Approach Shows Promise

Your exercise regimen may actually be more important for your brain than it is for your muscles, and the Maffetone Method (properly known as the "180 Formula") is the key to your brain's optimal efficiency.

Dr. Maffetone and I are good friends. I served as the Vice-President of the United States Chapter of the International College of Applied Kinesiology under his leadership. We worked closely together for several years and I learned a lot from him.

Dr. Maffetone is considered to be the king of aerobics. One of his patients ran over fifty miles each day—the equivalent of two marathons; he ran across the United States. This patient is so aerobically fit that he runs like the wind because he can. Another patient holds the record for the fastest 1,000-mile race. Dr. Maffetone treats many marathon runners, tri-athletes, and Ironman® participants. He knows what it takes to be aerobic and his patients are proof of his expertise. His method of calculating one's optimal aerobic heart rate is described as follows:

Movement and Exercise

Many people's nervous systems have had to adapt to an increased sedentary lifestyle, long hours spent viewing TV, and endless computer sessions at home and at work. No wonder there has been such a dramatic upswing in ADD/ADHD, autism, learning disabilities, and behavioral problems over the past twenty years. Many authorities have linked them to the appearance of TV and video recording media. Kids no longer move as much as they used to. Obesity and the consumption of junk foods are ever increasing among American children and adults.

Our bodies are designed to move. The human nervous system is designed to move in response to gravity. Reciprocal movement like exercise and sports is probably the largest contributor to proper human brain development and overall health.

Determining Your Optimal Aerobic Heart Rate

Subtract your age from a base heart rate of 180. Next, modify this number by selecting among the following categories the one that best matches your fitness and health profile:

> *Exercise may very well be more important for the brain than for the muscles.*

A. If you have or are recovering from a major illness (heart disease, any operation or hospital stay, etc.) or are on any regular medication, subtract an additional 10.

B. If you are injured, have regressed in training or competition, get more than two colds or bouts of flu per year, have allergies or asthma, or if you have been inconsistent or are just getting back into training, subtract an additional 5.

C. If you have been training consistently (at least four times weekly) for up to two years without any of the problems just mentioned, keep the number (180–age) the same.

D. If you have been training for more than two years without any of the problems listed above, and have made progress in competition without injury, add 5.

Then, subtract another 10 from this number to give you your ideal heart rate in beats per minute (bpm).

> *Exercise, when done without attention to neurological wellness contributes to functional dysfunction— deafferentation that results in cortical and cerebellar atrophy.*

Example: A thirty-year-old runner who has average health and occasional aches and pains for any reason, (fitting into letter B above) would train at a pace between 135 and 145 bpm. The math: 180-30=150; 150-5=145; 145-10=135. In this example, 145 would be the highest training rate. This is highly aerobic, allowing you to most efficiently build an aerobic base. The average person who works out at the upper end of this pace, or higher, has a very high probability of overtraining and doing it wrong. Training above this heart rate rapidly incorporates anaerobic function, evidenced by a shift to burning more sugar and less fat for fuel.

My own clinical experience with the 180 Formula shows that people usually exercise too hard. Dr. Maffetone believes that, "the heart rate is directly related to, and a reflection of, the body's oxygen need," and I

> *Exercise without considering its effects on the brain is like eating without regard for its effects on the tissues.*

would strongly agree. Any exercise routine that exceeds a person's functional capacity has a very high probability of causing muscle and joint breakdown that eventually leads to brain timing troubles. When patients follow the 180 Formula, they not only have more energy and enjoy better workouts, but they also have a nervous system that works as it should, according to its original and intended programming. That is what true health is all about—being healthy.

Is This You?

Ask yourself these questions: Do I feel good after my cardiovascular exercise? Does my heart rate jump right up to my target

It is a very important neurological rule that centerline structures work with centerline brain nuclei. There is no more centerline structure than the spine, and there is no more centerline nerve center than the thalamus. Therefore, it makes sense that the spine and thalamus work together. Whatever you do to one also affects the other. And if one breaks down, the other one breaks down also. Centerline structures are directly related.

rate? Do I sometimes go beyond my target rate just to work a bit harder? Does my heart rate get up to 150–160 beats per minute, and do I keep it there for fifteen to twenty minutes? Longer? Do I huff and puff a lot during exercise? Do I feel nauseated or feel like vomiting after I exercise? Do I start sweating right after I start exercising? Do I keep sweating even after my shower? Does my heart rate stay up for a while? Do I feel "a high" after exercising this hard?

While it is true that aerobic exercise is wonderful, more may not necessarily be better. If you answered "yes" to any one of these questions, *you may be setting yourself up for heart troubles.*

Aerobic Exercise

Aerobic exercise increases the demand for more oxygen and accelerates blood flow. The movements of exercise generate signals to the brain that come back to the heart and keep it from beating too fast. That is, exercise, when done according to your individual restrictions, keeps your heart rate constrained and within your own unique physiological limits.

The brain craves these incoming exercise signals—the highest priority of them coming from the muscles of the centerline spine—and the heart loves the safeguards they bring. In fact, because of the way that aerobic exercise builds endurance by improving mitochondrial performance and how the muscle's use stimulates the brain, it becomes clear that cardiovascular exercise may be more important for the brain than it is for the heart. Proper aerobic exercise stimulates a greater output of blood from the heart—the stroke volume—rather than increasing the heart's rate.

At a functional neurology seminar on human performance, the speaker examined a person who came up from the audience. The speaker calculated the person's optimal exercise heart rate using the 180 Formula, then examined the person to see the functional stability of their muscles. As is usual with most people, some muscles tested strong and others tested weak.

Next, the speaker asked the person to run around the room to quickly bring their heart rate into their target zone, and then come back onto the table. A subsequent exam showed that those muscles that had previously tested weak stayed weak, but those that had previously tested strong also became weak.

The person was given significant time to recover from the exertion, followed by another brief examination. The state of the muscles was again noted. The person was instructed to walk around the room for 10 to 15 minutes to slowly bring their heart rate into its target zone, and then to come back onto the table where they were examined again. The speaker found that not only did the previously strong muscles remain strong, but those muscles that previously tested weak also became strong.

This series of tests indicates that an appropriate warm up and cool down are an essential part of any exercise; they are as important as the right kind of exercise itself. Further, we realize that it takes time to functionally shunt blood from the organs to the periphery (the muscles) where it is needed during exercise. Jumping right to the target heart rate can be detrimental to the muscles and ultimately the brain, because that is the ultimate destination for the muscle input.

A healthy heart is one that stays within strict limits. Given average health status, the newest heart evidence indicates that an average forty-four-year-old female should keep her aerobic heart rate between 121–131 beats per minute. That is 30–33 beats every fifteen seconds. Does this sound too slow for you? Read on.

Revving your heart too fast can lead to trouble. Recent research shows that a heart attack is primarily an electrical event rather than solely the result of a blood clot.

It is theorized that a fast-beating heart can generate clots and therefore heart problems are more likely to occur. However, according to the *Brain Journal*, 2005, heart attacks appear to start in the brain and not necessarily in the heart, especially when the heart beats faster than the brain wants to allow. That leads to trouble.

The latest heart attack statistics prove more losses than gains. They show that women are more likely to die of a heart attack than of any other cause. Women are almost three times more likely to die of a heart attack than breast cancer. While men have more heart attacks, women "catch up" to men as they age. The blunt truth is that there is a very high probability that every person will eventually develop heart disease and it is only a matter of time until symptoms appear. Nobody wants a heart attack, but how many people are taking the proper care of their heart to prevent one?

Here is the point: An EKG checks the heart, but it cannot check the brain's ability to manage the heart. Most people exercise too hard and run the risk of becoming another heart attack statistic. They unknowingly unplug their heart from their brain and problems develop. Unhealthy heart habits are painless until that one fatal episode, and that means trouble. That is how heart disease got the name, "*the silent killer*."

The heart is a muscle. The stricter and more consistent you are with your heart rate, the greater the challenge it will be to reach your target range, and the healthier

While watching a stress EKG recently, I observed the 12 leads from the patient that were monitoring heart functions. The technician said, "You seem to be looking for something specific."

Actually, I was thinking that the EKG monitors heart function. While this is certainly necessary, there are many more aspects of heart function to monitor, such as the brain and how it is working.

Using one heart-related muscle, the heart-brain connection can be checked in 20 different functional ways. One author describes 17 different muscles that relate to heart function, so the math says that there are actually about 340 ways to check the heart and its relationship to the brain. All these tests are non-invasive and painless, and they can be used with the EKG to yield a more complete picture.

> *Endurance exercise can increase oxygen utilization from 10 to 20 times over the resting state. This greatly increases the generation of free radicals, prompting concern about enhanced damage to muscles and other tissues. The question that arises is, how effectively can athletes defend against the increased free radicals resulting from exercise? Do athletes need to take extra antioxidants?*
>
> *Because it is not possible to directly measure free radicals in the body, scientists have approached this question by measuring the by-products that result from free radical reactions. If the generation of free radicals exceeds the antioxidant defenses, then one would expect to see more of these by-products. These measurements have been performed in athletes under a variety of conditions.*
>
> *Several interesting concepts have emerged from these types of experimental studies. Regular physical exercise enhances the antioxidant defense system and protects against exercise induced free radical damage. This is an important finding because it shows how smart the body is about adapting to the demands of exercise. These changes occur slowly over time and appear to parallel other adaptations to exercise.*
>
> *On the other hand, intense exercise in untrained individuals overwhelms defenses resulting in increased free radical damage. Thus, the "weekend warrior" who is predominantly sedentary during the week but engages in vigorous bouts of exercise during the weekend may be doing more harm than good. To this end there are many factors that may determine whether exercise induced free radical damage occurs, including degree of conditioning of the athlete, intensity of exercise, and diet.*

your brain becomes. Read that last sentence again, it is *very* important. Aerobic exercise—when done properly—quickens the right kind of nerve signals from the muscles and joints and sends them straight to the brain. This switches on the systems that regulate heart rate. Broad-based aerobic control is crucial for proper heart health. Daily moderate exercise—within strict heart rate limits—not only builds heart muscle, but it also stimulates the brain and manages the heartbeat.

The threat of the dreaded "heart attack" can prompt many to turn their lives around. But why wait? Make changes now to help reduce your probability for heart disease and help you live a longer, healthier life.

We can tell if your heart is plugged into your brain. The test is simple and painless. If you have questions about the 180 Formula, please let me know. We can do the arithmetic together.

Summary

Breathe in, breathe out. Your brain is plastic—it can change. The brain can change relative to its environment; these changes can either be healthy or degenerative. Beneficial plasticity improves human performance, while detrimental plasticity breaks down cells and damages tissues leading to eventual deterioration and disease.

There are many ways to change a brain's plastic state. First, you can help it breathe better by keeping the Krebs cycle and electron transport chain active, ensuring that plenty of ATP is present.

Plasticity is aided by ensuring the availability of the ECRs in order to keep the cell membranes healthy. This means ingesting the right fatty acids, those that build the right structure that fits together just as it should and with no spaces between them. Avoiding trans fatty acids puts the right curves into the cell structure, and this helps signals and nutrients penetrate the cell membrane according to their original design.

We can help the brain work more efficiently by supplementing with certain herbs, vitamins, and minerals, as well as the right kind and amount of water for optimal cellular clarity.

Finally, the right kind of exercise is essential for a healthy brain. Remember, exercise may very well be more beneficial for the brain than it is for the muscles. While the muscles do the exercise, it is the brain that receives all input coming from the muscles and it had better be right. Any movement that is not according to the brain's original programming will cause chaotic working order, and this display will be obvious to a professional who is trained to see it.

People cannot recognize their own degenerative changes because they cannot perceive what the brain cannot receive, so it is hard to know when the brain is deteriorating (i.e., aging). You have the choice to influence your brain's plasticity one way or the other—for better or for worse. You can continue your old, unhealthy habits with their negative effects or you can put together some new regenerative habits that lead to health. It does not take long to produce an outcome, and with a few positive changes, you can feel better, quickly. That is why it is of vital importance to be treated by a Chiropractic Neurologist who uses applied kinesiology as functional neurology.

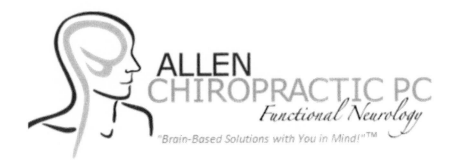

"Brain-Based Solutions with You in Mind!"™

SECTION II

"I CAN'T TAKE IT ANYMORE!"

CHAPTER SIX

IF YOUR BRAIN COULD SPEAK, IT MIGHT SAY...

"I Can't Take it Anymore!"

Although people are living longer, the prevalence of degenerative brain disorders is on the rise. While there is a wealth of information about having a healthy body and heart, there is little information about what it means to have a healthy brain.

> *When a person ages gracefully, they move and think with fluidity. Their thoughts and mannerisms are according to their original human design, and all their muscles have their proper display.*

A healthy brain means more than the ability to live a "normal" life. It is more than carrying on meaningful conversations, having a good memory, or using the right words in a sentence at the right time. All these are signs of a *functioning* brain, but are not the way to gauge a *healthy* brain; having a healthy brain means graceful aging.

If Your Brain Could Speak, What Might It Say?

In Section One, "I Can't Breathe!" we learned that the brain contains the most oxygen-sensitive tissue in the body. The slightest reduction in available oxygen to the brain has a profound impact on its performance. In

> The brain cannot survive too many toxins, incomplete nutrients, or the lingering byproducts of metabolism. Like all organs, the brain also must be clean to work its best.

Section Two of this book we will learn the importance of a healthy diet and what happens to the gut—and therefore the brain—when the diet lacks the essential nutrients for repair. If your brain could speak, it would probably say, "Quit doing this to me!"

The foods we eat are directly related to how our brains work. For example, many of the neurotransmitters essential for brain function come from, or are related to, the diet and gut. Generally, whatever is good for your body is good for your brain.

The nutrients from foods are broken down and reconnected in the gut, and then sent directly to the liver, and then on to nourish your cells. Some nutrients are transported directly to your brain, which either controls, produces or releases every hormone in your body. Simply put, if your gut has problems, then your brain will have problems. If nutrients cannot be digested properly, then there is no way the brain will get what it needs. The appropriate nutrients cannot be available if their source cannot be digested properly. When your brain has nutrient deficiencies, this means we can expect neurotransmitter trouble; the whole body suffers because the brain cannot work as it should.

> Gut problems are characteristically related to behavior issues and learning troubles.

A healthy population of friendly bacteria in the gut is fundamental to a healthy digestive tract. The digestive flora not only helps break down the contents of the digestive system, but they also stimulate the production of antibodies in the blood and enhance the immune system.

Friendly bacteria help produce substances such as Vitamins B and K, which are essential for overall health. They also help prevent infection from harmful bacteria, fungi, and parasites. Further, friendly flora produces natural antibiotics, acids, and hydrogen peroxide. In a sense, the normal digestive flora helps keep inflammation under

A Thought About pH

The pH of a fluid represents its level of acidity or alkalinity; it is either an acid or—it's chemically opposite—a base. The pH scale measures from 0 to 14, with a pH of 7 being neutral. Water has a pH of 7.

Importance of pH

Different systems have different pH levels. Saliva is almost neutral, while the pancreas needs a pH of about 8. However, to be healthy, the acidity of the stomach must be quite low.

Normally, stomach acid has a pH of 1 so it can break down everything eaten to prepare it for digestion. Proteins, for example, require a very low pH for their digestion in order to separate their amino acids properly.

As the stomach pH moves even one or two points toward neutral, it becomes less and less efficient, and this creates problems.

Reflux Issues

Stomach juices should have 1 million more hydrogen ions than water. But for every step toward neutral—from a pH of 1 to 2, for example—the stomach juices lose hydrogen ions by a factor of 10, or from 1 million times more acidic than water to 100,000 times more acidic than water. That may not seem like a lot to worry about, but when it comes to bloating, heartburn, or esophageal reflux each step away from where your pH belongs can be felt!

Antacids or acid-blocking medications—alkalizers—are not the answer to stomach symptoms because their alkalinity moves the stomach pH further away from where it works best, or else stops the acid production altogether. In fact, a reduced acidity—an increased alkalinity—is an excellent reason to add acidifiers rather than alkalizers. However, while taking some sort of acid supplement may be helpful, there are many other reasons for gastric troubles and they should be properly diagnosed. Good health begins in the gut.

control. If the populations of friendly bacteria get out of balance, those harmful organisms (called opportunists) take advantage and increase their ranks. Too many bacterial toxins increase the potential for inflammation and this means trouble—added stress for our digestive and immune systems.

Foods Are Our Best Medicine

The brain stem connects the brain and gut. An unhealthy brain can cause digestive problems, abnormal hormone levels, autoimmune disorders, allergies, and/or frequent sickness. The same can be said for an unhealthy gut.

> *One very good way to minimize inflammatory potential is to increase the presence of friendly bacteria. Ingesting pre- and probiotics tilts the scales in the favor of a healthy gut.*

One of the most common systemic insults people commit against themselves is eating foods that are nutritionally deficient. If your brain could speak, it might say, "Don't fill me with those calorie-rich belly bombs that contribute to my nutrient deficit." A well-balanced diet, which includes antioxidants from whole foods, is best.

> *If your brain could speak, it would probably say that it needs to be taken care of better!*

"Non-foods" fill the shelves of most grocery stores, but they should never pass for food. They are full of additives to enhance their taste and prolong their shelf life. In many cases these additives increase the appetite and suppress the sense of fullness, leading to cravings, obesity and sickness. No wonder diabetes is on the rise.

Keep reading. The more you understand, the clearer you will see what you can do to reduce your toxic load and build a healthier brain.

Good Digestive Function is Vital

The "best" diet is useless in the presence of digestive issues and ultimately leads to malnutrition and functional brain problems. Since the human brain governs all human functions, any dysfunction there will negatively affect all aspects of its host.

Improving the human brain function requires adequate digestion and dietary modifications. Reduced carbohydrate intake, adequate consumption of essential fatty acids and essential protein combined with a healthy digestive tract help create the biochemical basis for optimal brain function.

Process This: The Truth about Commercial Foods

Philosophers have pondered this event called life since it first began. Their ideas about physiology boil down to the term "homeostasis." Homeostasis (*homoios*, "similar" and *stasis*, "standing still") is the physiological processes necessary for life to persist. It is a sensitive balancing act between the different but interdependent factors responsible for sustaining the normal events of life.

There are three key components necessary for life. Each depends on its balance with the other two. One aspect has to do with the sensory *input* from

> *Isomers are compounds with the same chemical formula, but different structures.*

muscles, organs, digestion, air, sensations, and other information we receive from our environment. Another part is a *monitor* of all the input, and the third part is the motor *response* to all that input. The point: In most homeostatic mechanisms—those physiological pathways that make all systems work according to their original plan—the control center is the brain. *The brain determines the fitting response to various stimuli.* The appropriateness of the response is directly related to the health of the brain, and that response can be measured.

The brain's internal environment is quite sensitive to its surroundings. Its activities are swirlingly busy, yet highly ordered. Nerve tissues and other cells that surround the nerves need oxygen, glucose, basic nutrients, and water before they can work efficiently. If any of these essential components for brain health are missing—or if there is too much of a substance that should not be present—it can reduce your ability to learn and/or function at your highest levels. In some cases, even the slightest changes can negatively alter homeostasis possibly even ending life itself. However, ensuring your brain has a good and available supply of all these building blocks provides a solid foundation upon which the other parts of the brain can perform well.

> *Trans-fats may have been outlawed in many foods and restaurants, but they are still created—they still become hydrogenated—every time oil is heated in the open frying pan or skillet.*

These days, we must all be very careful of what we take into our bodies. Most people know that junk food is bad. Fried foods, simple sugars, and low nutrient quality may be very tasty, but they are very dangerous to good health. What about those foods that are supposedly "healthy"? How about those fruits and vegetables that appear to be good for you but are actually full of toxic surprises? Many seemingly healthy foods are grown in soil full of pesticides and sprayed with chemicals that have unpronounceable names.

There is a field near the freeway in Oceanside, California, where food crops are grown. It often seems that driving by it most likely requires a gas mask because of the blatant pesticides in use. The same is—or at least it used to be—true when driving through many areas of Irvine or California's central valley. Foods contain the substances found in the soil in which they are grown, and they absorb what is on them. Further, many fruits and vegetables are irradiated before they reach the grocery shelves. In their raw state, these crops are thought to be nutritious and good for you, but the catch is in their processing. For example, during their processing, many foods get a wax covering to slow the food's dehydration and make them shinier, and more appealing.

Foods that would have been previously good for you now have many potential toxins added to them. Besides pesticides, many otherwise good foods are all too often tainted with dyes, preservatives, trans-fats, high-fructose corn syrup, and other additives that make them full of flavor, yet full of undesirable consequences. If your brain could speak, it would probably say, "Treat me right!"

Brain Fat Is Not Body Fat

A Carbon Atom with Four Available Bonding Sites

Somewhere along the road to health, the important things all got changed around. Fats have always been good for us but now we are told that fats make us fat. People over-respond by assuming *all* fat is bad, and they eliminate all fats from their diet believing it will help them stay thin or lose weight. We are so concerned with our weight! We drink soda pop laden with sugar or sugar substitutes, eat pasta and bread, cookies and cakes. And we wonder why our waistlines keep expanding. The truth is that simple carbs and the stuff in them make us fat. If your brain could speak, it would probably say, "I want the good stuff, eliminate the bad!"

Did you know that a major portion of our brain contains fat? Fats surround the nerves, making up the nerve's protective sheath; it's the nerve's insulation. Fat is essential for healthy nerves. Without a proper amount of fat the human nervous system misfires, it's prone to injury and it is more easily damaged. This low fat craze has damaged the nervous systems of many adults and children.

Trans-Fats

It is important to understand carbon's chemistry a bit better. Please do not get turned off by the word chemistry because this is fun. Trans-fat is the common name for unsaturated fats with *trans*-isomer fatty acid(s). As we previously discussed in Chapter Five, trans-fats may be mono-unsaturated or poly-unsaturated, but never saturated.

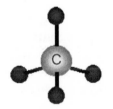

A Carbon Atom with its Four Bonding Sites Filled by Hydrogen Atoms

Carbon Atoms

Each atom has a certain number of slots for other atoms to attach to it. For example, sodium has one and calcium has two. A carbon atom has four slots available for other atoms to attach to it. The slots are called bonding sites. Those sites can be used for just about any other atom that will bond with it.

How Unsaturated Fats Got Their Name

Even in a long chain fatty acid, there are still only four possible bonding sites per carbon atom, but in most cases one site on each carbon atom is used to connect to another carbon atom—one carbon on each side of the bond, the bond taking up one site on each carbon atom. That leaves two other available bonding sites for each carbon, each for a hydrogen atom, for example.

$$R\!-\!\overset{\displaystyle |}{C}\!=\!\overset{\displaystyle |}{C}\!-\!R$$

An Example of an Unsaturated Bond, where "R" Represents the Rest of the Chain

When carbon atoms are double-bonded to each other, there are only two other available bonding sites—one for another carbon and one for another molecule because carbons can only have a total of four bonds. In a generic fatty acid, hydrogen might take up those sites, so there are fewer hydrogen atoms in an unsaturated molecule than in a saturated molecule, hence the double bond is said to be "unsaturated." If that double bond broke, it would become singularly-bonded, or saturated.

As we have seen, the terms "*cis*" and "*trans*" refer to the arrangement of chains of carbon atoms across the double bond. Recall that in the *cis* arrangement, the hydrogen atoms are on the same side of the double bond, resulting in a kink. In the *trans* arrangement, the hydrogen atoms are on opposite sides of the double bond, and the chain is straight.

> A new study out of the University of Alberta (UA) in Canada clarifies a common misunderstanding about trans-fats—natural, health-promoting, ruminant trans-fats [those fats from pasture-based cows, sheep, and goats that are present in organic meat, milk and other dairy produce; mostly the main 'natural' monounsaturated trans-fat vaccenic acid, which can be metabolized by humans to conjugated linoleic acid (CLA)] are far different from the synthetic, health-destroying, industrial trans-fats resulting from hydrogenation and commonly found in many processed foods.
>
> Their study showed that these naturally occurring trans-fats have a vastly different fatty acid profile than industrial trans-fats like hydrogenated vegetable oil. This does not mean that all the trans fatty acids are in themselves harmless, but that any harmful effect is limited and balanced by the beneficial effects of, for example, trans isomers of conjugated linoleic acid (CLA) which are health-promoting with specific physiological roles.
>
> The natural trans-fats can actually help reduce the risk of developing cardiovascular disease and cancer, while industrial trans-fats found in various processed foods lead to conditions like high cholesterol and coronary heart disease.

How Hydrogenated Fats Got Their Name

A fat becomes hydrogenated when hydrogen gas is injected into *cis*-unsaturated fats in the presence of heat. That eliminates the double bond (or bonds) and "saturates" the bonding sites with hydrogen atoms (i.e., heating an unsaturated oil makes it hydrogenated), converting them into indigestible trans-fatty acids that are far worse than natural saturated fats could ever be.

Food manufracturers prefer hydrogenated fats because they have a higher melting point and an extended shelf life. They can be found in

> I recently asked the manager of a well-known local fast food outlet how often they change their French fry oil, and they said every two weeks.

Hydrogenated and partially hydrogenated fats are known to raise "bad" cholesterol levels.

restaurant foods, fast foods (French fries, fried chicken, and chicken nuggets), snack food, packaged bakery products (cookies, crackers, donuts, breads, and cakes), microwave popcorn, potato chips, peanut butters, and salad dressings.

Fast food outlets seem to take great pride in touting their "no trans-fat" use of food preparation. While they may use trans-fat-free oils in their preparation, once heated the damage is done. Remember

Here is a good rule when it comes to trans-fats: Stay away!

that it is high heat and oxygen that "hydrogenate" the oil, changing the *cis* form of the molecule into its unhealthier trans-type. Fries, for example, are usually cooked at about 375°F for four to five minutes, but techniques vary depending on the method used. French fries have about 40% trans-fat, and many cookies and crackers range from 30 to 50% trans-fat. Donuts often have up to 35% trans-fats.

Trans-fats cannot be properly metabolized in the human body because their molecular shape keeps them from being recognized by digestive enzymes. Remember, trans-fats have straight chains and *cis*-fats are curved. Enzymes know the difference and they build tissues accordingly.

Half-Life

The term "half-life" is used to measure the length of time it takes for half of a substance to be eliminated. The term was originally used to describe how long it took for a radioactive substance to decrease by half, but it can be used relative to any substance that breaks down or dissipates. The half-life of trans-fats is about fifty-two days. That means that it takes almost two months for half of the consumed trans-fats to be gone. Since the foods you eat make up every component of the cells of your body—every part, from the cell membrane to the nu-

The half-life is the time it takes for half of a substance to break down. The half-life for a given item is independent of how much of that item you consume or how long it has been sitting around.

Being Careful of Fats

With the exception of only a few oils that can withstand high temperatures, the essential fatty acids are very susceptible to heat, light, and oxygen, which destroy the bonds and straighten out the kinky chains. Flaxseed oil is quite susceptible to the effects of heat, so it should not be used for cooking. So when consuming foods for their essential fatty acid content, it is a good idea to avoid cooking or heating them. For example, it is better to eat raw nuts than to eat roasted nuts. Finally, do not reuse any type of oil. This is a common practice when making fried foods like French fries—just ask the cooks sometime.

Many health enthusiasts believe that hydrogenated fats are unfit for human consumption and they should be replaced right away. California was to be the first state (AB 97, 2008) to have eliminated trans-fats from commercial foods. Remember, the half-life of hydrogenated fats is about fifty-two days, taking them almost two months to eliminate half of them from your system.

Many people use a small amount of ground flaxseed on their vegetables. It adds those essential fatty acids that make healthy membranes and other vital components, and adds a nutty taste. Adding whole flaxseeds will not do the same thing. The cells of the seeds must be thoroughly macerated to release the oil, but neither the human teeth nor digestive system can do that. Therefore, the flaxseeds themselves usually pass through your digestive system whole, absorbing water but not yielding much oil.

If you use vegetable shortening, replace it with half as much virgin olive oil and a pinch of salt in a salad, in the frying pan, or in a recipe.

Many supermarket salad oils are full of additives and metabolites that tend to clog your system. So adding ground flaxseed and/or virgin olive oil to salad is another healthy change.

Replace oily snack foods, like potato chips, French fries, and corn chips, with nuts and seeds.

cleus itself—two months after consuming trans-fat, half of the amount eaten is still wreaking havoc with your tissues, making them do things that they were not designed to do, or not do things they were designed to do, simply by virtue of their altered structure. In the next two months, half of

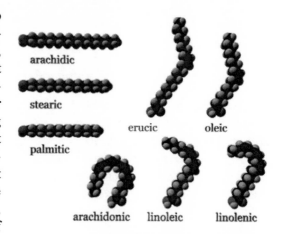

Fatty acids of various shapes are important for cell membrane integrity

what was left is still there. In another two months, half again is lost but 12-1/2% of that trans-fat eaten about six months previously still remains in your cells. Arithmetically, some residual trans-fats always remain in your tissues once they are consumed.

Unlike good fats, trans-fats are not essential to good health, in fact, just the opposite is true: they are toxic.

Several studies have shown that eating non-food fats increases one's risk of coronary heart disease. The health community agrees that the consumption of trans-fats must be eliminated if people want good health. Trans or hydrogenated fats from any source are contrary to good health.

In pregnant women, just as alcohol, drugs, pesticides, and carbon monoxide from cigarette smoke pass through the placenta to the baby, so too do trans-fats. Fetal tissues grow faster than at any other period in that person's lifetime. These tissues are ravenous for the building blocks of good health, and they are affected in direct proportion to the amount of trans-fats eaten by the mother. Because they are growing so quickly, a developing baby's tissues are more sensitive to this onslaught of toxic insult than adult-sized tissues. Before the baby takes its first breath, its tissues may have already been damaged by toxic assault. In addition, there is a correlation between trans-fats and Type 2 Diabetes.

Empty Calories

Many research projects have proven that one of the greatest health dangers is consuming too many empty calories. In fact, eating these simple carbohydrates can help accelerate age-related brain changes.

Simple carbohydrates are toxic to nerve cells. Diabetes is the primary example of what happens to the nervous system when blood sugar levels are too high. The nerves actually die. You end up with diabetic neuropathies that lead to the amputation of limbs.

Reactive hypoglycemia—blood sugar that falls too low as a result of dietary error—is equally dangerous. Many people on high carbohydrate diets suffer from dramatic blood sugar swings. The brain and the peripheral nervous system require an even and constant supply of glucose. When blood sugar levels drop too low, too fast, neurons are unable to function properly. They become stressed and may actually die off.

In order to improve brain and nervous system function, it is thus vital to reduce carbohydrate intake, especially sugar.

Sadly, there is mounting evidence that suggests that simple carbs offered by the food manufracturing industry has created obesity, diabetes, and many of the other chronic degenerative diseases seen today. Food colorings, dyes, additives, and preservatives are not found in natural foods. Foods in their natural state have all the necessary ingredients needed for their digestion and assimilation, but the demands of an "I've-got-to-have-it-now" marketplace keep us from considering the costs of a nutrient depleted diet.

Eating nutrient-rich foods in their natural state may slow your biological clock and maintain your youthful vitality. Be sure the foods you eat are nutrient-dense to get as much out of your calories as pos-

> *Check out the GRAS (Generally Regarded as Safe) list. It is an excellent way to see what is allowed in the American diet!*

sible. Empty calories and simple carbs can actually accelerate aging because they lack the vital nutrients that keep tissues strong and healthy. If your brain could speak, it would probably say, "Quit treating me this way!"

Processed "Foods"

> ### *An Apple*
>
> *Start with seed.*
>
> *Because "I am an 'original food'," let ripen on tree; pick.*
>
> *Please note: Food in its original state. "If nobody eats me, I will ripen anyway, preparing myself for new trees."*
>
> *"You're welcome."*

Processed, pre-packaged foods have almost completely taken over the American foodscape. The industry estimates that nearly 90% of American's food budget is spent on processed foods. Many of the most common foods are processed or have been modified from their natural state in order to feed the masses. They tend to have multiple additives to extend their shelf life. Across an entire fast-food menu, there are thousands of ingredients, ranging from the commonplace (water) to the exotic (xanthan gum).

Unfortunately, most healthy foods are transformed into some other substance for consumption—by humans or animals—either in the home or by the food processing industry. These processes typically take clean, harvested crops or butchered animal products and use them to produce attractive, marketable and long shelf-life food products. This is similar to the processes used to produce animal feed. These "foods" are laden with sweeteners, salts, artificial flavors, factory-created fats, colorings, chemicals that alter texture, and preservatives. Examples of such foods would be ice cream, margarine, and even dog food. Another example would be those foods that contain GMOs, but the food manufracturers are not required to put any identifying ingredients on the label, making the public's consumption of such "foods" a guessing game.

For the first time in history, the Food and Drug Administration (FDA) is considering the approval of genetically engineered fish for sale and consumption in the United States. Not only does this raise tremendous concern about the safety of the food, but also of the

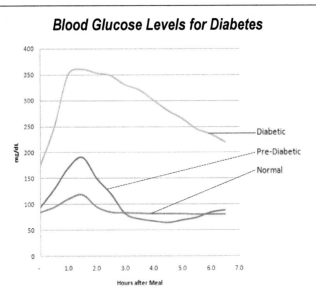

Blood Glucose Levels for Diabetes

Your brain runs on a steady supply of blood sugar, converting an incredible 20% of the carbohydrates you consume for energy. Simple carbohydrates and sugary foods cause unpredictable blood sugar highs and lows, with a rush of sugar into the bloodstream. These wild swings trigger an insulin response meant to manage the blood sugar. If these blood sugar swings are not controlled by a specific sequence of organs, the blood sugar level crashes, leading to hypoglycemia. For example, low blood sugar causes the release of adrenal hormones, producing a "sugar high" that squeezes stored sugar from the liver, sending blood sugar levels back up again.

These blood sugar swings create a roller coaster effect, with "sugar highs" and "sugar blues." The ups and downs of blood sugar and adrenal hormones can also stimulate neurotransmitter imbalance, causing you to feel fidgety, irritable, inattentive, panicky and even sleepy. This is not the most beneficial state for efficient brain function. Since simple carbohydrates have been implicated in diabetes as well, you may want to think twice before eating simple carbohydrates or sugary foods.

food chain in general. Aqua Bounty Technologies has created a genetically modified salmon, trout, and tilapia; the genetically modified Atlantic salmon is the first of the applications, the end result is being nicknamed *"Frankenfish"* because the product is so heinous. However, documents released by the FDA staff state that the altered salmon are "as safe to eat as food from other Atlantic salmon." The agency said it found "no biologically relevant differences" in vitamins, minerals, or fatty acids.

Butter versus Margarine

In the U.S. butter must contain at least 80% butter fat with the remainder made up of water and milk solids.

Margarine makers start with cheap, poor quality vegetable oils, such as corn, cottonseed, soybean, safflower seed and canola, and then add:

- *Veggie-oil blend*
- *Water*
- *Whey (milk)*
- *Salt*
- *Veggie mono & diglycerides*
- *Soy lecithin*
- *Citric acid*
- *Artificial flavors*
- *Vitamin A*
- *Beta carotene (for color)*

But the problem is not just what's been added to foods, but it is also what has been taken away. The processing of foods often strips away the specific nutrients that nature intends to protect us from sickness. Soluble fiber, antioxidants, and "good" dietary fats are all essential components for cellular and tissue repair, without which those tissues cannot be strong. Combine that with additives, and you have a recipe for disaster. White flour and pasteurized dairy products have both been heavily processed, removing essential nutrients meant to enhance the health of the original products. The original whole wheat product is stripped of its mineral content and a few of the essential nutrients are added back again. Pasteurization of dairy products denatures proteins and renders almost half of the calcium unavailable for digestion. Neither "food" is fit for human consumption.

Some items on market shelves should not be classified as "food." Processed meats, NutriSweet® (Equal®, Aspartame®, and most recently Acesulfame potassium, also known as "Acesulfame K®"

---

or "Ace K®"—K being the symbol for potassium—and marketed under the trade names Sunett® and Sweet One®), pickles and salt-cured foods, colas and sodas, artificial coloring, caramel coloring, (homogenized) milk, rancid oils, and processed sugar can also contribute to health problems. They will not kill you or make you sick right away, but the signs and symptoms of sickness are a gradual process. Your risks of sickness and disease increase as these non-foods are consumed over time.

Aqua Bounty's mission is to have a major role in "The Blue Revolution"—the convergence of biological sciences and molecular technology, with the goal to advance the aquaculture industry, enabling large-scale, efficient, and environmentally sustainable production of high-quality seafood. According to Aqua Bounty, "increased growth rates, enhanced resistance to disease, better food-conversion rates, manageable breeding cycles, and more efficient use of aquatic production systems are all important components of sustainable aquaculture industry of the future."

Colorings, Dyes, Additives, and Preservatives

People like consistency in their foods and nature has satisfied our desire for "eye candy." When oranges are allowed to ripen naturally, its nutrients are higher; it looks appealing, smells appealing, and feels appetizing. However, mass marketing changed all this around. Society has been trained to think that certain colors should taste a certain way. People associate colors with flavors, and they want their foods to be a certain color.

Today's foods must be picked before they are ready to be separated from their source and left to mature en route, but a food's maturation does not equal its nourishment. Just like any other

Food dyes have been linked to kidney tumors in mice, brain gliomas in male rats, urinary bladder and testicle tumors in rats, thyroid and adrenal cancers in animals, hypersensitivity (allergy-like) reactions in some consumers and may trigger hyperactivity in children.

Chapter Six: "I Can't Take it Anymore!" • **173**

biological process, the end stage of ripening requires certain nutrients that cannot be available once the food is separated from its source, whether it is on a tree, a bush, a vine, or a root. Enter the food dyes and artificial chemicals that manufracturers add to fool your eye into believing food's appearance—it's only skin deep. Oranges are all made to look the same color orange and they taste orange, and cherries are all made to look the same color red and they taste red. Who wants to eat a brown orange or a green cherry?

> *Some people may have physical reactions to these substances. Look for natural coloring agents like turmeric, paprika, or saffron instead.*

Seasonal changes, soil variations, processing techniques, and storage procedures can affect the color of foods, so adding color adds consistency, uniformity, and familiarity, making foods taste as expected based on their ingredients. While most shoppers know that green catsup, for example, or Magic Stars® cereal are likely colored, few people know that apples and salmon are sometimes dyed to mask natural variations in color.

In their natural state, biochemical processes naturally break foods down into their component parts. Bacteria, fungi, and/or antioxidants bring about natural chemical changes in color and appearance, but that hinders profits, so commerce stepped in to slow the breakdown by adding preservatives and additives.

There are not many rules to regulate the use of food colorings or dyes. Food manufracturers are allowed to use as much food dye as necessary for them to achieve the color they desire. However, it is hard to find any research that details the half-life of a food dye. The quest to find out "how long does the most widely-used and consumed food dye— red dye #40, or Allura Red—stay in the human system" is unresolved. The same is true for other food colorings. No one knows how long it takes to eliminate the negative effects of food dyes.

A Recipe for Disaster

1 part Trans-fats
1 part Favorite Food Coloring
1 cup Rancid Oil

Process above in the lab, wrap in colorful plastic, attach catchy name. Let sit on shelf for 2 months. Now eat it.

The Real Cost

Most health-conscious people shun preservatives, additives, food colorings, flavorings, and dyes. However, as newer and potentially dangerous flavor enhancers and other additives find their way into our foods fewer people know how to recognize them. Sometimes there are so many chemicals added to food that it becomes impossible to keep them all straight. These potentially dangerous ingredients may even have several different names, requiring the general public's constant vigilance. For example, there is a great deal of controversy regarding the dangers of food dyes and colorings. Particular groups have been shown to be sensitive to these additives, which reportedly trigger headaches, tingling, abnormal behaviors (such as isolation and aggression), and other symptoms. Older studies were apparently unable to draw any conclusive evidence linking food dyes and colors with ADD, but newer studies point to synthetic preservatives and artificial coloring agents as aggravating ADD and ADHD symptoms, both in those affected by these disorders and in the general population.

> *Natamycin is used in the food industry as a "natural" preservative. Natamycin (also known as pimaricin and sometimes sold as Natacyn) is a naturally occurring antifungal agent. Natamycin is effective at very low levels. It is classified as a macrolide polyene antifungal and, as a drug, is used to treat fungal keratitis. Other common members of the polyene macrolide antifungal family are amphotericin B, nystatin, and filipin.*

Preservatives are aptly named because they keep foods and pharmaceuticals from breaking down. Calcium propionate, sodium nitrate, sodium nitrite, sulfites (sulfur dioxide, sodium bisulfite, potassium hydrogen sulfite, etc.), and disodium EDTA are just a few of the more common anti-microbial preservatives. The commonly found BHA (butylated hydroxyanisole) and BHT (butylated hydroxytoluene) are antioxidant preservatives. Many chemicals and additives are the subject of debate among food academics and regulators specializing in food science and toxicology, and of course biology; what else is food science except biology.

Many of the modern synthetic preservatives have been linked to respiratory and other health problems, and this causes controversy regarding their usefulness. According to some studies, ADD, ADHD and other problems related to learning have been linked to synthet-

Seitan® is made from the gluten of wheat, being called "wheat meat" or "wheat gluten," but it actually has little in common with flour or bread. It is also simply called "gluten." While it is high in protein and popular with vegetarians, it is toxic to many people with gluten allergies.

ic preservatives. At the same time, other studies have shown that removing artificial ingredients from school food programs reduced the incidence of disciplinary problems and enhanced the academic performance of school aged children. But despite the growing controversy, food companies continue using synthetic ingredients to manufacture these non-foods, and people keep eating them without fully realizing the dangerous physiological consequences of their choices both now and down the road.

Common Additives that Raise Serious Health Concerns

Too much or not enough of any substance can lead to disease. Metabolic pathways are like rivers. They should flow freely from one end of the pathway to the other. Flow limitation means back up; like a dam that impedes progress, metabolic restrictions limit free flow. Providing the essential components for repair of a pathway does two things: it blows the dam and frees the flow.

Considering that some of these potentially dangerous ingredients have been implicated as the cause of serious health issues, it would be good to know which of these are the most common. According to the U.S. Food and Drug Administration, the most common of those additives are:

Gluten: It is a baking agent commonly referred to on the packaging as a protein. Gluten adds to the elasticity and color of the finished food product and functions as a stabilizing or thickening agent. Many products will not say specifically that they contain gluten, but will use "wheat syrup" and "malt" as the most common gluten-based additives.

Gluten is a common ingredient in vegetarian and vegan cuisine, appearing as wheat gluten. Meat substitutes contain seitan®, a cooked and flavored form of gluten that mimics the texture of chicken, steak, and other meats. It can also be added to broths as a protein and thickener. Chewing gum, ice cream, catsup, and many candies contain gluten.

Gluten can be very toxic to the human brain. In fact, 80% of Caucasians are sensitive to the protein (gluten) in wheat. It can cause bloating and a sense of fullness in the gut and that can lead to digestive errors that impact the ability to make many of the neurotransmitters that involve the brain.

Like many other items we ingest, gluten has its own characteristic half-life. According to the Gluten Free Society, gluten antibodies typically have a half-life of three to four months—that is 90 to 120 days. Thus, it takes that long to eliminate half your gluten response from your body. It takes another three to four months for half of what is left to be eliminated, and so forth until the gluten is metabolized. This is all considering that there is no new gluten consumption from hidden or accidental sources. However, the truth is that according to this scenario, gluten antibodies are statistically never completely eliminated once they appear.

Gluten's breakdown depends upon several other factors. For example, gluten-induced liver and/or kidney issues—which are quite common in gluten sensitivity—can prolong the process of gluten's removal. Another complicating factor is the persistent intake of sometimes even the smallest amounts of gluten, which increases inflammation and muddles the immune response. The level of hydration also plays a roll in gluten's detoxification; dehydration slows the detoxification process. Constipation is also an issue because slowed gut motility complicates gluten's removal.

However, gluten metabolism can be enhanced by supplementing the diet with enzymes that break down foreign proteins and their metabolites, nutrients to help the stomach produce hydrochloric acid, and pre-

and probiotics for immune support. Together, these issues make unraveling liver and kidney involvements—and any other related problems—essential to treating gluten-sensitivity.

> Gluten can wreak havoc in the human nervous system.

<u>Citric acid</u>: the most common preservative. While citric acid is considered a natural product that is essential to the Krebs cycle, too much of it can put an unnecessary load on the tissues to handle it. An added burden exists when the Krebs cycle dysfunctions because of nutrient deficiencies.

<u>High-fructose corn syrup</u> (HFCS): virtually unknown prior to 1966, it has become the most common sweetener and a very popular food additive; not popular because people want it, but for its usage. People want the sweetness it provides—an inexpensive liquid six times sweeter than cane sugar—and its manufracturers like the fact that HFCS is cheaper, significantly sweeter, and easier to transport, and that it is a simpler to use alternative to regular sugar, but few know of its dangers.

> The consumption of high fructose corn syrup (HFCS) in the U.S. has increased by a whopping 10,700 percent between 1970 and 2005.
>
> —the USDA Dietary Assessment of Major Trends in U.S. Food Consumption report.

HFCS accounts for more than half of the entire sweetener market bringing its manufracturers over $4 billion in sales each year. And consumption continues to grow. According to the U.S. Department of Agriculture, in 2011, the average American consumed more than forty pounds of HFCS per year from processed foods, including soft drinks, condiments, applesauce, and baby food, (up from zero in 1966). Recent studies show that on average, people consume about twelve teaspoons of HFCS per day, while teens and other high consumers ingest 80% more HFCS than average.

Research indicates that HFCS may be one of the most implicated causes of obesity. Although it is essentially sugar, it has replaced white sugar as the sweetener of choice in many beverages and foods such as breads, cereals, breakfast bars, lunchmeats, yogurts, soups, and condiments. It is made by subjecting corn syrup to an enzymatic process that increases its fructose level.

Many researchers have begun to question the relationship between HFCS in foods and obesity rates in the United States since it was introduced to food producers over four decades ago. Some critics believe that HFCS is more dangerous to health than table sugar (sucrose). Proponents claim that the low cost of HFCS encourages manufacturers to use it in food preparation, and consumers to eat more of it.

MSG has been known to cause an extreme rise or drop in blood pressure, arrhythmias (irregular heartbeat), depression, dizziness, anxiety or panic attacks, migraines, mental confusion, stiffness, muscular swelling, lethargy, seizures, joint pain, flu-like body aches, chest pains, loss of balance, slurred speech, diarrhea, stomach cramps, sneezing, nausea, vomiting, skin rashes, hives, blurred vision, and difficulty in concentrating.

In addition to its relationship to obesity, HFCS has been implicated in high levels of mercury. One recent study found that almost half of tested samples of commercial HFCS contained the heavy metal. Further, high mercury levels were also found in nearly a third of fifty-five popular brand-name foods and beverages where HFCS is the first or second highest labeled ingredient.

Caramel color: one of the oldest and most widely-used food coloring additives. It is found in almost every kind of industrially produced food, from batters and beers, to brown breads and buns; from chocolate to cookies, and from brandy to whisky. Caramel color can be found in desserts, fillings and toppings, potato chips, dessert mixes, donuts, fish and shellfish spreads, frozen desserts, fruit preserves, glucose tablets, brown gravy, ice cream, pickles, sauces and dressings, soft drinks (especially colas), cookies and pastries, vinegar, and wines.

The international food community has limited the daily intake of caramel color relative to body weight, but the FDA has not acted accordingly. It appears that the FDA believes that unless there are

> The percentage of vital minerals in different salts varies greatly from one natural salt to another. Even within the same salt farm installation, it is possible to extract two salts of slightly different magnesium content.

known problems with caramel coloring, food manufractuders may use it however they like. That means in the US, we may be getting more caramel coloring in our diets than our bodies can handle.

Some research has found that caramel coloring may be toxic, carcinogenic, or mutagenic—having the potential to change genetic material, usually DNA. It has also been found that caramel coloring can potentially lead to intestinal problems, but the International Programme on Chemical Safety oversight group "says" they have found no evidence.

Some caramel colorings come from maize, which has a high probability of being genetically modified. However, that genetic modification cannot be detected by standard procedures.

Finally, after its processing, caramel coloring can retain traces of sulfites. But the finished product does not need to note any sulfite levels above ten parts per million on the food label.

> MSG is used as a salt-substitute and flavor enhancer. This additive is found in many processed foods, as well as restaurant prepared foods.

Salt: the most common flavor or spice. Added salt is a major contributor to high blood pressure. Sodium can hide in the most ordinary foods, like sauces, soups, and baked goods. Most people know that eating too much sodium can contribute to long-term health problems, but most are unaware that it can also cause fluid retention and bloating.

Reduce your salt intake by opting for fresh foods and the low-sodium versions of products, including condiments like salad dressing, ketchup, and mustard. Take the salt shaker off the table and use herbs instead of salt for seasoning. Some people prefer salt that is less processed, like sea salt. But regardless of what type of salt you use, healthy adults should only consume between 1500 to 2300 mg of salt per day.

<u>Monosodium glutamate</u> (MSG): found in almost all convenience foods, fast foods and processed foods. It is the most common flavor enhancer of cheap, processed foods to try to make their taste more appealing. MSG comes from the processed remains from boiling soy, corn, or wheat in hydrochloric acid. The residual is a brown powder—hydrolyzed vegetable protein, or HVP—that contains large amounts of glutamic acid, which consumers are more familiar with as monosodium glutamate, or MSG—glutamic acid's one-sodium salt.

MSG by any name is just as toxic. It is an excellent example of a stealthy toxin unfit for human consumption, yet people continue to disregard the seriousness of its threat. Much literature links MSG with ADD, ADHD, obesity, and many other brain-related sicknesses.

> *There is a loophole in the legislated food labeling laws. If the free glutamate or glutamic acid is less than 78% of an additive, it doesn't have to be labeled MSG. That means that 75% free glutamate is legal without notice.*

MSG appears to have dozens of aliases that disguise its presence. Among them are: any enzyme-modified ingredients, autolyzed yeast, autolyzed yeast extract, autolyzed yeast protein, calcium caseinate, flavoring, flavors, gelatin, glutamate, glutamic acid, hydrolyzed corn, hydrolyzed plant protein (HPP), mono-potassium glutamate, natrium glutamate, so-called "natural" flavors, sodium caseinate, spices, textured protein, ultra-pasteurized, yeast extract, yeast food, or yeast nutrient, and the list goes on and on. Many manufacturers of medications use MSG as a filler ingredient in tablets and other medications. Even personal care products like shampoos, soaps and cosmetics contain MSG. Look for ingredients that include the words "hydrolyzed," "protein" and "amino acids." The point is that MSG is often hidden behind seemingly familiar terms. To keep your health, you must understand what you read on food labels—*caveat emptor.*

> *There seems to be considerable debate about MSG's beginnings. Apparently, the FDA's procedures were questionable and MSG's health issues remain unanswered. Nonetheless, it is a good practice to stay far away from MSG.*

MSG is an excitotoxin. It kills nerve cells fast by accelerating their aging, making them swell up and *POP* in a split second!

In an attempt to make bland foods taste more appealing, this chemically structured ingredient has been linked to neurotransmitter damage and the weight gain problems we see today. Researchers suspect that MSG's toxic effects are more dangerous to the hypothalamus. They believe that MSG affects the appetite control centers there, which has led to the increased commonness of obesity. *People sensitive to MSG should avoid eating any substance that contains MSG's aliases.*

> *Unless they are vigilant, restaurant owners may be unwittingly exposing their patrons to MSG. The food industry uses many different disguises for labeling sauces and dressings, for example, which contain free glutamates.*

HVP is one of the worst of the MSG line of offenders. Another name for HVP is "vegetable protein" or "plant protein," and besides glutamate, HVP contains high levels of the excitatory amino acids aspartate and cysteic acid—an intermediate in cysteine metabolism.

The FDA has failed to protect consumers from the dangers that MSG poses to their health, having found its way into protein powders, prepared foods, diet products, cereals, frozen dinners, sauce mixes, soups, salad dressings, and many other manufactured food products. Even so-called "natural" seasoning and spices can be 12 to 40% MSG.

Many unhealthy additives can slip past an unwitting consumer. Reading food labels is an art that many people just do not have unless they have taken biochemistry classes. Is that unawareness a good thing? With regards to knowing what we ingest, definitely not. Many of the words on a food label may relate to common food items, but that does not mean they are good for you. By law, food labels are to clearly reveal the packaged contents. But as we have seen, MSG, for example, can be disguised by many different names, so it may not be obvious to the untrained eye.

Two other common toxic ingredients in many foods are calcium caseinate and soy protein isolates. To many people, these two ingredients may be as dangerous as MSG. Calcium caseinate is a tasteless, odorless, water-soluble, white powder that is used in emulsification and stabilization. It is formed by dissolving casein (milk protein) in sodium hydroxide and then evaporating it, leaving casein sodium or nutrose.

Niacin: the most common nutrient in foods. It is one of the many fractions of the B complex, found in beverages, cereals, biscuits, cakes, desserts, egg and cheese dishes, fats and oils, fish and other seafood, fruits, meats and meat products, milk and milk products, nuts, sauces and condiments, soups, sugars, jams and spreads, sweets, and vegetables. While niacin is a B-vitamin, its individual presence can cause stress in peripheral tissues, eventually depleting those tissues of the nutrients they need to perform their own functions.

Soybean oil: the most common oil or fat in foods. Products containing both liquid and partially hydrogenated soybean oils are exported abroad, sold as "vegetable oil" or end up in a wide variety of processed foods. Soybean oil does not contain the EPA or DHA fatty acids, yet it does contain a significantly greater amount of omega-6 fatty acids. One hundred grams of soybean oil contains 51 grams of omega-6 fatty acids, and 7 grams of omega-3 fatty acids. That is just over a 7:1 ratio (of omega-6 to omega-3 fatty acids). As a comparison, flaxseed oil has an omega-6:omega-3 ratio of 1:3. Soy also contains substances that mimic estrogen, possibly leading

A higher ratio of omega-6 fatty acids can be found in most types of vegetable oil.

to endocrine problems. Some researchers might disagree with the postmenopausal and endocrine finding, so this debate is unsettled. Hence, soybean oil continues to make its way into the food supply.

Mono- and diglycerides: the most common food emulsifiers. Simply, mono- and diglycerides are fats, usually derived from soybean, cottonseed, sunflower, or palm oil. They generally keep baked products from getting stale. Mono- and diglycerides can be found in ice cream and other processed foods, including margarine, instant potatoes, and chewing gum to give them body and improve their consistency.

The 8 most common food allergens:

- Gluten
- Milk
- Eggs
- Fish
- Peanuts
- Shellfish
- Soy
- Tree nuts such as almonds or cashews

But mono- and diglycerides are almost always on lists of questionable foods for people with celiac disease—a lifelong digestive disorder—because of the possibility that wheat might be the carrier for their usage. However, the FDA apparently has no food label requirements that convey a particular outcome because their content is usually negligible by the FDA's definition.

However, the Food Allergy Issues Alliance (a group of food trade associations and consumer interest groups who are concerned about food allergens) recently encouraged the FDA to warn food manufracturers that the eight most common food allergens should be included on food labels. This should at least allow the consumer to make an educated food choice.

Xanthan gum: the most common food stabilizer or thickener; it slows the flow of liquids. Xanthan gum is the product of the bacteria-related fermentation of two sugars—glucose and sucrose. However, while some xanthan gum is not derived from corn, these bacteria are sometimes *fed corn* to help them grow, causing some people to display an allergic reaction to xanthan gum.

Some people are more sensitive to xanthan gum than others. One study concludes that xanthan gum has a laxative effect, producing symptoms of intestinal grippes and diarrhea. But there are no studies yet investigating whether or not this is considered to be an allergic reaction. There are even reports that some workers exposed to xanthan gum dust developed respiratory complaints.

Chicken: the most common meat product. As a food, chicken has been depicted in Babylonian carvings dating back to around 600 BC. It was the most available meat in the middle ages. It is considered easily digestible and one of the most neutral foods.

Chickens that are raised in close confinement—called factory farming—are routinely fed a compound that decomposes into an inorganic arsenic compound, which is more toxic because it is in its unbound form, and can be detected in their skin and feces, but not in their meat. However, this compound did show up in potentially dangerous amounts in chicken livers. This issue is apparently watched closely by the FDA, who says their samples apparently show far less arsenic than would otherwise be allowed in a food product for human consumption.

Four Common Processed Food Additives

Rats that were fed a diet high in trans-fats showed fundamentally abnormal changes in that area of the brain responsible for learning and memory.

Trans-fats: the artificially produced fats used in margarine and many processed foods. At first they appeared to be even worse than saturated fat when it comes to clogging arteries. Partially hydrogenated oil may also be listed as an ingredient. Now, alarming new studies indicate that these same fats are considered to also "gum up" our brains. As a result, product labels are now required to list the amount of *trans* fat in a serving.

The new alarm was triggered by Lotta Granholm, director of the Center on Aging at the Medical University of South Carolina, who did a six week experiment in which rats were fed a diet containing trans-fats—either soybean oil, which is unsaturated, or partially hydrogenated coconut oil, a commonly used trans-fat. Next, researchers put the rats in a water-filled maze to test how well the rats could

> *Trans-fats are made when heated oils are exposed to the air. That "hydrogenates" the bonds. Any food made with hydrogenated or partially hydrogenated oil contains trans-fats.*

recall the location of submerged platforms. Rats usually dislike swimming, so they were highly motivated to find relief. The reluctant rats on the trans-fat diet took significantly longer to find these platforms than those rats on a regular diet and made many more mistakes during the test.

The scientists later studied the rats' brains and were surprised to find abnormally formed proteins in the hippocampus (a part of the brain that is important for learning and memory) of the rats on the high-trans-fat diet. "The kind of damage we saw may make it harder for brain cells to create the connections required to build memories," says Granholm. "What's especially troubling is that these animals ate amounts of trans-fats proportionally similar to what many people consume."

Despite the presence of these deformed proteins, the scientists were at a loss to determine how they got there. They considered that it may be related to the presence of zinc and copper used to solidify the trans-fats at room temperature. Although both of these metals are critical to health, high levels of zinc and copper have been found in patients with Alzheimer's disease. Rats fed trans-fats also showed signs of undue inflammation, which could damage brain-related proteins.

Experts say that this news underscores the importance of avoiding trans-fats, which have been conclusively linked to hardening of the arteries, or atherosclerosis. While there are increasing calls for their elimination altogether, the FDA indicates that they will require trans-fats to be listed on food la-

> *Removing the germ and bran from the rest of the grain essentially separates the life-giving parts from the food, making it an incomplete material.*

bels. It is reported that after watching her rats floundering in a water maze, Granholm immediately went home and emptied her refrigerator of all foods that had partially hydrogenated oils or trans-fats listed on the label.

Foods for a Healthy Brain

Healthy foods lead to healthy tissues, and unhealthy products lead to a sick brain. Your brain will demonstrate its health relative to the items you choose to include in your diet.

Fruits

Acai berries	Avocados	Bananas	Blueberries
Cantaloupe	Cherries	Cranberries	Oranges
	Raspberries	Tomatoes	

Vegetables

Broccoli	Cauliflower	Brussels sprouts	Peas
Collard greens	Potatoes	Romaine lettuce	Spinach
	Red cabbage	Soybeans	

Seeds

Almonds   Walnuts*

Nuts

Cashews   Walnuts*

Grains

Oatmeal

Other items

Cheese	Chicken	Eggs	Fish/fish oils
Flaxseed oil	Legumes	Milk	Olive oil
Peanut butter	Real chocolate	Salmon	Tuna (in water)
Turkey	Water	Wheat germ	Yogurt

* Walnuts are seeds, not true nuts.

Refined grains: refined grains are generally referred to as those grains or grain flours that have been significantly modified from their natural—whole grain—composition by mechanical removal of bran and germ, either through grinding or selective sifting. They are further refined by mixing, bleaching, and combining the material with bromine or a bromine compound—a process called bromi-nating. Then the process adds back the previously stolen B-vitamin fractions—thiamin, riboflavin, niacin—and iron to "nutritionally enrich" the product. Because the added nutrients represent only a fraction of the known nutrients removed, refined grains are considered nutritionally inferior to whole grains.

<u>Salt</u>: the overconsumption of refined salt is known to increase the risk of many health problems, including high blood pressure. Natural or unrefined salts contain all four positively charged electrolytes (sodium, potassium, magnesium, and calcium) as well as other vital minerals needed for optimal bodily function, like iodine, manganese, boron, copper, silicon, iron, and nickel. And it is these other vital minerals that make all the difference. Not only are they essential for optimal health, but their proportions are important for certain biochemical processes to occur. For example, if potassium is in excess in relation to sodium, the body's enzyme pathway loses its ability to produce hydrochloric acid. So if we have to use salt, chose natural or unrefined sources.

Eating too much salt over a long period of time is associated with increased risk of stroke and cardiovascular disease, muscle cramps, dizziness, and electrolyte disturbance, which can cause neurological problems and even death. However, some scientists believe that excess salt intake has no significant role in hypertension and coronary heart disease, as they believe adults' kidneys are able to remove excess salt. On the other hand, drinking too much water, with insufficient salt intake, puts a person at risk of water intoxication, or hyponatremia.

The risk for disease due to insufficient or excessive salt intake varies because of our biochemical individuality. Evidence supports the link between excess salt consumption and heartburn, osteoporosis, hypertension, left ventricular hypertrophy, edema, duodenal ulcers, and even death in the case of the ingestion of a large amount of salt over a short period of time.

<u>High-fructose corn syrup</u> makes the list again. It is the fourth of the most common ingredients in processed foods. Any surprise? It is in almost anything you buy from a grocery store.

Nine Inedible-Sounding Food Additives

<u>Polydimethylsiloxane</u> (PDMS; a silicon-related compound also known as dimethicone): a food additive used as an anti-foaming and anti-caking agent. It has been reported to be added to many processed foods such as McDonald's Chicken Selects® Premium Breast Strips, and many other fast food items.

<u>Carrageenan</u>: a common additive that is extracted from seaweed. It is used in ice creams, soy milk, toothpastes, patés, diet sodas, and even beer. It is often used externally to resemble streaks of fat in lean meat marbling, as well as in shampoo, shoe polish, pet food, and in personal lubricants.

A recent publication indicated that carrageenan may produce inflammation in the human intestinal tract leading to possible bowel disease. Some studies indicate that carrageenan that is broken down by high temperature and acidity may cause gastrointestinal ulcerations or cancers. It also reportedly interferes with immune function.

<u>Monosodium glutamate</u> (MSG): glutamate is also known as the "umami" flavor, considered to be the fifth "essential" flavor detectable by the human palate (the others are salty, sour, sweet, and bitter). As discussed previously, MSG (glutamate with an added sodium atom) can cause some pretty nasty side effects for sensitive people.

<u>Phosphoric acid</u>: a corrosive material more commonly known as the substance that gives soda its acidity and sharper flavor. It is also used in fuel cells, to remove hard-water stains, and as a pH balancer in cosmetics.

In some studies, the phosphoric acid used in many soft drinks has been linked to lower bone density. However, there appears to be lots of controversy regarding phosphoric acid in sodas. One recent study in the *American Journal of Clinical*

> *The respiratory cycles of plants exchange carbon dioxide for oxygen while those of mammals exchange oxygen for carbon dioxide. These two processes are at the center of life itself.*

Nutrition that was based on x-ray studies rather than questionnaires about breakage, provided reasonable evidence to support the theory that drinking colas can lead to lower bone density.

However, Pepsi® funded its own study that indicated that the *insufficient intake of phosphorus* could lead to lower bone density. Really? (I bet you are wondering if you read that right; you did.) Then again, the study did not examine the digestive effect of phosphoric acid. Instead, they focused on the general phosphorus intake. Phosphorus tends to bind with magnesium and calcium in the digestive tract to form salts that are not absorbed.

Finally, other "controlled studies" have shown that there is no relationship between phosphoric acid and bone calcium loss, even when compared to water, milk, and various soft drinks—two with caffeine and two without caffeine, two with phosphoric acid, and two with citric acid.

Sorbitol: when consumed in mass quantities, acts as a laxative. It is found in sugar free mints, medicines, gums, and diet sodas. It can also be found in make-up, mouthwash, toothpaste, and even in some cigarettes.

Gelatin: collagen extracted from the bones, connective tissues, organs, and some intestines of domesticated cattle, pigs, and horses. It may be used as a stabilizer, thickener, or texturizer in foods like jams, cream cheese, and margarine. It is found in some "gummy" candies as well as other products such as marshmallows, gelatin dessert, trifles, confectioneries such as Peeps® and Jelly Babies®, and some low-fat yogurt.

Since gelatin comes from cattle, some concern exists about the spread of animal diseases, like mad cow disease, or Bovine Spongiform Encephalopathy (BSE). However, the FDA and other agencies say that they constantly monitor and minimize the potential risks. All reputable gelatin manufacturers today follow strict guidelines to ensure that their products are consumable.

Xanthan gum: contains bacteria similar to rotting vegetables. Think of it as that film that forms over molding veggies. Then it is easy to understand how xanthan gum thickens those ingredients used in manufactured food products, such as dairy products, sauces and salad dressings.

Carmine: a bright red food coloring agent; from the primarily sessile—or basically immoveable—scaled parasite, commonly known as the cochineal. Carmine consists of a mixture of crushed beetles. They are boiled in water to extract their carminic acid, and used to artificially dye foods red, purple, and pink. It is found in some fruit juices, berry punches, ice cream, yogurt, and candy.

Some people have shown an allergic reaction to carmine, including a mild case of hives, atrial fibrillation, or anaphylactic shock. Some people have symptoms of asthma, and hyperactive children should stay away from manufactured foods with carmine. In 2011, when used as a food additive the FDA required that carmine be listed on food labels

High-fructose corn syrup makes the list again. Despite its popularity, an argument can be made that HFCS may be one of the big reasons behind the growing obesity epidemic. Sweetness is a preferred and acquired taste that may be enhanced by exposure to sweet foods.

Beware: Toxic Metals

Consider the foods that contain fatty acids, amino acids, and micronutrients. They all seem to contain the nutrients necessary to benefit the system as a whole. That is, the result of their interactions is greater than the sum of their individual effects. When these individual whole molecules are separated—as when fatty acids are hydrolyzed, or the amino acids are denatured, or when the micronutrients are split—the individual aspects of the whole nutrients are incapable of nourishing our bodies as nature intended when naturally blended. They have certain abilities when they are in their whole form, but these abilities are not the same when the natural molecule is fractionated, or split into its separate parts. This segregation can expose the molecular pieces to toxic metals—such as mercury, lead, nickel, arsenic, and cadmium—that relocate to the slots where the molecules came apart.

> *People often tell me that they drink green juices like wheat grass to give themselves more oxygen. While that may be the end result, it is not exactly what happens.*
>
> *Wheat grass juice—by virtue of the chlorophyll it contains—binds carbon dioxide, contributing to tissue detoxification while at the same time allowing for hemoglobin to drop off the oxygen necessary for proper tissue metabolism.*

Chlorophyll is a complex molecule much like hemoglobin. Chlorophyll is the pigment in vegetables that makes them green and it is involved in transforming the sun's energy to energy that we can use for food. Hemoglobin is responsible for binding oxygen and transferring it to our tissues. In general, chlorophyll is to plant cells what hemoglobin is to mammal red blood cells.

At the center of their structure, chlorophyll and hemoglobin are essentially the same. There are some bonding differences, but generally, chlorophyll has magnesium at its center and hemoglobin has iron. While chlorophyll binds to carbon dioxide and releases oxygen, hemoglobin binds to oxygen and releases carbon dioxide.

Chlorophyllins—a water-soluble semi-synthetic salt derivative of chlorophyll—are made by removing the magnesium from the center of a chlorophyll molecule and replacing it with a copper atom and

> *Some say chlorophyllins are potentially toxic when used internally because of the copper they contain.*

adding a sodium atom on the chlorophyll molecule's periphery. This ever so slight substitution makes the molecule different, and that changes the way it works. Instead of taking chlorophyllins internally, they can be used as a skin wash useful for both treatment and odor control of wounds, injuries, and other skin conditions—notably radiation burns—and are potentially toxic to the liver.

Toxic Metals in Our Foods

Toxic metals can easily make their way into the foods we eat. Overall, today's foods are more toxic than they were even twenty to thirty years ago. Their toxicity does not necessarily appear in themselves, but in the way they are used in the body. Trans-fats, for example, have come under fire because of their relationship to heart disease. Although trans-fats help increase the shelf life of foods, these same foods become unhealthy when the trans-fats are added.

> *Environmental chemicals—xenobiotics—have an overwhelming effect on the brain's timing centers. They are called "endocrine disruptors" because they interfere with sensitive systems like NTs, NCs, and hormones. They can cause developmental disorders, including learning disabilities, severe attention deficit disorder, cognitive and brain development problems. Any system in the body controlled by hormones can be derailed by hormone disruptors.*

Scientists from Dartmouth University have tracked five potentially toxic heavy metals—arsenic, mercury, cadmium, strontium, and lead—as they climb the aquatic food chains and ultimately into the human body. Toxic metals are dangerous because they can imitate the action of essential nutrients, disrupting the metabolic processes and ultimately causing illness. Arsenic interferes with sulfur and many enzyme systems; mercury interferes with nitrogen, oxygen, sulfur, and selenium; cadmium interferes with zinc; strontium and lead interfere with calcium, and the list goes on. Tissues, bones, enzyme systems—like those that detoxify the liver—and immune processes are all susceptible to toxic metal assault. We need to be aware that even small changes to food components—for whatever reason—have giant repercussions. Are you listening? Your brain is.

Most alarmingly, some of the latest data indicates that mercury may be found in high-fructose corn syrup. Sadly, rather than asking which foods contain high-fructose corn syrup, a shorter list can be obtained by asking for foods that *do not* have it. High-fructose corn syrup can be found in just about every food on grocery store shelves.

Medical journals are chock full of articles about how the brain changes. As we have discussed, the brain wants to change—this is called plasticity and the brain changes relative to its stimulation. Appropriate stimulation can lead to healthy brain function but unnatural stimulation can produce faulty behavior. It all has to do with the result of brain stimulation—plasticity. While we once thought that brain function was unchangeable, we now know that it is easily influenced by what we do to it; by the toxicities we subject it to.

Aluminum is another toxic metal that can damage the human brain. It comes in through several seemingly innocuous paths, like cookware, foil, antacids, deodorants, and toothpastes; we call these xenobiotics—external sources of toxic exposure.

Exchanging heavy metals for the naturally found minerals of a vitamin complex changes how that vitamin complex does its work. The wrong metal in a chemical equation or genetic sequence can lead to a devastating process that would otherwise have been under nature's perfect control.

Food Irradiation

 or

**Treated with
irradiation**

**Treated by
irradiation**

The Logos for Irradiated Foods. Since 1986, all irradiated products must carry the international symbol called a radura. (Notice the subtle differences in the two pictures; "treated with" relative to "treated by" irradiation.)

The Radiation Information Network from Idaho State University states that irradiated foods provide the same benefits as those that are processed by heat, refrigeration and/or freezing; or are treated with chemicals to destroy insects, fungi, and bacteria that cause food to spoil or cause humans disease. They say irradiating food not only extends its shelf life, but it also keeps it in better condition in warehouses and homes.

However, there is another perspective. The simple process of irradiating foods, in an effort to destroy microorganisms, viruses, bacteria, or insects, also prevents sprouting, and delays ripening. In other words, irradiating food halts the natural growth processes.

Irradiating foods exposes them to a tremendous amount of high electromagnetic energy that causes an atom or molecule to change its electron pattern, taking on a change in existence consisting of perhaps one neutron; enough to change the molecular behavior. Ingestion of such foods could be dangerous if consumed by people, but not because it contains any radiation; it does not.

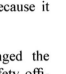

No Irradiation

Independent studies have challenged the claims by the FDA's own food safety officials who say irradiated foods are safe, despite the fact that irradiating foods can produce a molecule called furan—a known carcinogen found most often in thermally processed foods. FDA officials testified before Congress that the quantity of furan produced by putting x-rays through food was negligible. However, past research has shown that high doses of ionizing radiation can induce the formation of furan in solutions of simple sugars and ascorbic acid.

> *Reportedly, the U.S. Food and Drug Administration (FDA) is examining health concerns related to levels of the carcinogenic toxin furan in soy protein isolate and other foods.*

While some say irradiation can cause a change in texture, taste, and nutritional content of food—especially at the doses required to reduce pathogen levels so that the foods are deemed "safe" to eat—irradiation proponents say that an irradiated apple, for example, will still be crisp and juicy. Using ionizing radiation, they say, does not significantly increase a food's temperature or change the physical characteristics of most foods.

Until recently, the only irradiated foodstuffs marketed in the United States were dried spices and enzymes. Now, Florida strawberries and poultry have been added to the list.

> *Though most irradiated food sold in stores must be labeled, there is no such requirement for restaurants, schools, hospitals, nursing homes and other institutional settings.*

As in the pasteurization of milk (which is not the same as irradiating food), the irradiation process greatly reduces but does not eliminate all bacteria. Irradiated poultry, for example, still requires refrigeration, but would be safe longer than untreated poultry. Strawberries that have been irradiated will last two to three weeks in the refrigerator compared to only a few days for untreated strawberries because their "life" is gone. While pasteurization and irradiation are completely separate processes, neither one adds anything healthy to the foods in the common food chain. In fact, in the end the food is lifeless.

Potential Food Irradiation Uses

Types of food	Food Industry Benefits	Harmful Residual Effects
Meat, poultry	Destroys pathogenic fish organisms, such as Salmonella, Campylobacter, and Trichinae	There is a high probability that residual products of pathogenic organisms remain in the food
Perishable foods	Delays spoilage; delays ripening avocados; retards mold growth; reduces number of micro-organisms	Foods spoil when enzymes are present in the foods—that's life; delayed spoilage means fewer enzymes and less life
Grain, fruit	Controls insect infestation in vegetables, dehydrated fruit, spices and seasonings	Food attracts insects to participate in the food's breakdown; rips at the core of the nutrients
Onions, carrots, potatoes, garlic, ginger	Inhibits sprouting	Sprouting is a sign of life; no sprouts, no life in the food
Bananas, mangos, papayas, guavas, other non-citrus fruits	Reduces rehydration time	Delayed ripening means damage to the organic processes

[In the United States, the Food and Drug Administration (FDA) has approved irradiation for eliminating insects from wheat, potatoes, flour, spices, tea, fruits, and vegetables.]

There is questionable safety putting any food item through an airline security system that uses either x-rays or microwaves.

Nutritionists encourage people to increase their daily servings of fruits and vegetables because they contain antioxidants—the molecules that fight the free radicals that cause oxidation and cell damage. However, how can foods provide antioxidant protections if the "tools" we are given—irradiated foods—contain the very toxins we are trying so desperately to avoid!

It is said that during irradiation, the energy waves affect unwanted organisms but are not retained in the food. That may be true. Ionizing radiation can be harmless if it passes right through the food. The harm comes when the cellular components of the irradiated food are struck by the x-rays themselves. It is one thing if the primary or strongest x-rays get through the food, but what about any scatter? Scattered x-rays can be more dangerous than the original insulting irradiation be-

Neurotransmitters are brain chemicals that relay information. Their deficiency can negatively impact your personality, moods, relationships, and your overall experience of life. It can also impact how well functional neurology treatments work for you, making a neurotransmitter deficiency an important area to address.

cause their wavelength changes. Scattered x-rays are more readily absorbed by the substance they enter.

Let's Not Split Molecules

The point here is that ionizing radiation has the potential to split molecules apart. This separation generates free radicals, which quickly recombine, sometimes into unnatural or even harmful radiolytic—a known toxic particle—compounds. A good example of a radiolytic compound is 2-dodecylcyclobutanone (2-DCB), which is formed by the radiolysis of palmitic acid and is present at low parts-per-million levels in irradiated meat products.

Ionizing irradiation has been approved for many uses in about thirty-six countries, but that does not make it healthy for you. However, only a few applications are currently underway because of con-

In general, those products that hurt the brain also harm heart function. So stay away from these things if you want your brain (and heart) to be healthy.

- *Alcohol*
- *Artificial food colorings*
- *Artificial sweeteners*
- *Colas (diet and regular)*
- *Corn syrup (and high-fructose corn syrup)*
- *Cereals and cereal bars*
- *Deep fried foods*
- *Energy drinks*
- *Frostings*
- *High-sugar "drinks"*
- *Highly-greasy foods*
- *Hydrogenated fats*
- *Junk sugars*
- *MSG (and its related names)*
- *Nicotine*
- *Overeating*
- *Partially hydrogenated fats*
- *Processed foods*
- *White sugar*
- *White bread (and other white flour products)*

sumer concern and because the facilities are expensive to build. So far, the FDA has approved irradiation for eliminating insects from wheat, potatoes, flour, spices, tea, fruits, and vegetables. Approval was given in 1985 to use irradiation on pork to control trichinosis, and in 1990 to control Salmonella and other harmful bacteria in chicken, turkey, and other fresh and frozen uncooked poultry.

But the concern remains that if irradiation can affect insects, it can affect the substances in the food. Furthermore, and perhaps even more importantly, if irradiation does indeed kill these organisms, then it must leave the residue of dead insects and bacteria inside the food or on its surface. Not only is this an unpleasant thought, the residue may be toxic if it contains free radicals. Try not to worry about this too much—at least the residue is sterile.

Irradiation also can be used to keep sprouting and ripening under control. Consider this: if sprouting or ripening can be stopped, then the irradiation must have been successful. And that also means that the natural processes have been silenced and the food itself is dead.

Cooking with Microwaves

Insofar as the microwaves—which are not the same as x-rays—are concerned, cooking with microwaves is not recommended any more than eating irradiated foods. While microwave ovens do not use the same ionizing radiation as x-rays, the power of microwaves is well known to disrupt the fatty acids in the bounding cell membranes and alter their molecular structure, and potentially creating free radicals. So while no microwave radiation may be detectable inside the foods, the footprints that microwaves may leave in the cellular membrane are obvious.

Greater Nutrition in Live Foods

One of the first things I learned during my professional education was that a healthy diet should be 85% raw and 15% cooked. Raw foods provide many of the essential components necessary for tissue repair, like enzymes and micronutrients that are so important for many of the digestive processes. These foods are more nutrient-dense. Cooking food tends to eliminate these enzymes because they are so heat sensitive, and that reduces that food's quality.

Another important rule is to never miss a meal. Frequent smaller nutrient-dense meals are the key to eliminating drastic swings of blood sugar. Eat small helpings of fresh foods during the day to maintain that feeling of being satisfied, and eat it in a stress-free way; avoid eating on the run. This rule is one that I try to follow to this day.

People tend to consume extra calories when essential nutrients are missing from their diet. That is, they eat more when their foods are nutrient-poor. What could have been an efficient digestive system suffers when the essential components for nourishment and repair are missing, being replaced with increased calories. These extra calories in a nutrient deficient diet take the place of more beneficial foods, and the byproducts of their metabolism tends to congest the cells and tissues that work so hard. The building blocks of health cannot perform well with a diet void of adequate nutrition.

Whole and live foods ensure an adequate supply of the micronutrients—enzymes, vitamins, minerals, etc—that nerve tissues need to function well.

Brain Tips

Your brain needs a constant environment for optimal function: frequent small meals, plenty of oxygen, the right amino acid and neurotransmitter balance, the right micronutrients, and plenty of water.

Frequent Square Meals

If you give your brain the right nutrients, you will tend to think quicker, have a better memory with an improved ability to focus. Because the whole system is nourished better, you may also tend to be better coordinated and balanced.

While studies have shown the importance of a good breakfast, most people tend to sacrifice this one meal. After all, that is where the

> *Here is the best brain tip: Avoid processed food stuff!*

word "breakfast" comes from—to break a fast. It is the first meal you eat after sleeping—fasting—for six to ten (or however many hours you sleep) hours nightly.

Instead, many go for a cup of coffee or a sugar drink and a pastry from the local coffee shop. Breakfast should be the main meal of your day, the foundation upon which the rest of the day is set. It should consist of complete proteins, complex carbohydrates, healthy fats and oils, and it should be eaten slowly. Hurrying through breakfast defeats its benefits. Make yourself take the time to enjoy the start of every day.

Try to eat a protein-based lunch to optimize your mental performance and alertness throughout the day. Stay away from simple carbohydrates no matter how quickly you know they will increase your blood sugar. That boost will only drop you in a few short hours. These energy drinks will only be harmful in the long run.

> *Protein "isolates" are proteins that have been stripped away from their nutritional cofactors, presenting three potential problems. First, all isolates are detached from their whole food making them harder to digest and more acid forming. Second, the human system has a very hard time processing protein isolates, causing nausea, vomiting, bloating, constipation, and other complaints. Finally, because of over-processing, there is a high probability that protein isolates are deficient in their essential amino acids and nutritional cofactors.*

Dinner should be small yet packed with live foods. Salads, complex carbs, oils, seeds, and nuts will help you be ready for bed and sleep. Eating right throughout the day will set up the normal rhythms that encourage healthy body processes.

Take Time to Breathe

Some blood sugar issues may respond best to more frequent, small meals every day. Think back. Do you remember that we discussed how oxygen is the most essential component of brain health? Oxygenate your brain by exercising and keep your blood sugar constant by eating small meals more often. Three square meals a day may be too long to wait for someone whose blood sugar wavers like the breakers on a beach. Be sure to eat breakfast every morning, your lunch on time and without stress, and your dinner before seven p.m.

Some basic nutrients help control the way oxygen works. For example, fatty acids help oxygen build a strong brain, amino acids help the brain centers connect, and micronutrients protect the brain from many types of breakdown. This is the only way we should "be smart" about food, not irradiating it, processing it, adulterating it, and preserving it.

Thinking is a Biochemical Process

Proteins are made up of long chains of various amino acids. As a general rule of nature, protein-rich foods are naturally linked with fatty acids, indicating that nature intends that they should work together. Their blending with various vitamins and minerals is essential for developing brains, memory, and learning. Further, blending fats and proteins slows the uptake of the proteins, ensuring their more complete absorption.

> *Neurons carry electrical signals from one synapse to the next. They let related areas know what each other are doing.*

Our brains store longer-term memories in the many connections between neurons, called synapses, which are rich in special signal-carrying neurochemicals known as neurotransmitters.

While an electrical signal naturally flows through each neuron, there must be some way to get the signal from the end of one nerve to the beginning of the next. Neurotransmitters are that bridge (see the table, Neurotransmitters: Their Functions and Levels, pages 229 and 235). They relay the nerve signal from nerve to nerve, some passing on the signal and others quieting it.

The key here is timing; it all comes down to how one signal slips through a nerve center relative to another one; which one slips through first. While the nerve connections make long-term memories possible, it is the *timing* between the connections that creates long-term memory.

> *The essential—or indispensable—amino acids for humans are phenylalanine, histidine, isoleucine, leucine, lysine, methionine, threonine, tryptophane and valine. Under certain circumstances, the body is unable to synthesize arginine, cysteine, proline, serine, glutamine, glycine and tyrosine, making them conditionally essential.*

Thinking is a biochemical process; a primary result of nerve stimulation. The way neurons and nerve signals work together all comes down to timing. It is like an engine, the pistons and the timing chain. Using an automobile engine as an example: it is the timing chain that brings the pistons to the right place when the spark plugs fire. That means the engine will work smoothly and quietly. However, if the timing chain slips, then the spark plug fires before the piston is in the right place, and the engine knocks. The same idea happens in the human tissues. Muscles respond with integrity when their nerve signals are timed right. However, nerve signal timing errors create neurological static and the muscles work contrary to their original programming; they "turn off" when they should be "on," and are "turned on" when they should be "off."

The foods you eat have a direct effect on the performance of your brain because thinking takes linking. Fitting bits of neurological information together into meaningful biochemical blends is what generates memories. Connecting these bits requires "brain foods" like fresh fish, which is a rich source of both protein and fat. Meat, eggs, cheese and yogurt, grains, legumes, seeds, and nuts also contain

> *Diet, lifestyle, and general health greatly affect neurotransmitter activity. For instance, diets high in sugars and starches, as well as chronic inflammation or hormonal imbalances, can deplete key neurotransmitters. Functional neurologists address the cause of the deficiency or poor activity by using specific therapeutic activities and nutritional compounds to boost neurotransmitter activity.*

the amino acid building blocks and associated fatty acids necessary to make neurotransmitters. You can be sure to get your essential (also known as indispensible) amino acids and fats from a healthy protein supplement and eat right for the rest of your nutrients.

> *Every vitamin contains one or more of the particular minerals that make it work. Their functions are naturally inseparable.*

One special neurotransmitter is Acetylcholine (ACh); special because it is involved in so many physiological functions. It excites other neurons and may be responsible for memory. ACh is involved with voluntary movement of muscles, controlling behaviors, thinking, and memory. People with Alzheimer's dementia may have less ACh than someone with a neuro-typical brain or the available ACh is blocked for some reason. Acetylcholine rich foods include egg yolks, peanuts, wheat germ, liver, meat, fish, milk, cheese, and vegetables—especially broccoli, cabbage, and cauliflower.

Dopamine is responsible for feelings of pleasure and satisfaction, as well as muscle control and function. It generally excites the nerves,

As a general rule, if a person is deficient in an individual B vitamin factor, taking that individual factor may be the right way to treat it, but they should quickly transition to the entire vitamin B complex once that individual deficiency is resolved.

and is involved in movement, attention and learning, and emotional arousal, but it can also quiet nerve function.

People with Parkinson's disease (PD) may have a dopamine deficiency because the cells that produce it are either burned out or damaged causing a tremor that is noticeable when the furthest part of the extremities (most often the hands) are at rest. Slowness of movement, rigidity of muscles, and postural instability are also symptoms of PD. This is an example of how giving dopamine medicines can quiet the nerves, but that may not be the best remedy. People with these challenges can benefit by finding some way to increase their dopamine levels. Increased joint motion has also been shown to help.

Schizophrenia is associated with excess dopamine, as are digestive problems. Many children who appear to be slow to learn tend to show dopamine issues as do kids with developmental delay. Today, many of these issues can be found with a simple saliva lab test, and the results can lead to an alleviation of the problems. Further, since dopamine has so much to do with brain function, balancing dopamine levels can even change how a person perceives the world and their behavior.

In February, 1992, the *Archives of Neurology* had an article in support of the muscle/movement hypothesis in PD. It said that there appears to be a functional breakdown between

One pasteurization process raises the temperature of milk to 71.7°C (161°F) for 15–20 seconds and then immediately cools it after it is removed from the heat. This process theoretically slows spoilage, but it also denatures proteins and breaks down enzymes, makes fats rancid and renders more than 50% of the calcium unusable. Ultra-high temperature pasteurization holds the milk at a temperature of 135°C (275°F) for a minimum of one second. A less conventional but US FDA-legal alternative (typically for home pasteurization) is to heat milk at 145 °F (63 °C) for 30 minutes.

the usual power of movement that comes from muscles and joints and those that ultimately reach the brain. This dysfunction can lead to Parkinsonian-like symptoms and the characteristic depletion of dopamine that brings about the Parkinson's display.

Dopamine is made from the amino acids found in all protein foods, like meat, milk products, fish, beans, nuts, and soy products. As little as three to four ounces (about 85-115 grams) of protein a day will help you to feel energized, more alert, and more assertive. However, not all protein sources are equal, and not all people are able to use the protein they consume.

In 1993, the Food and Drug Administration and the Food and Agricultural Organization of the United Nations/World Health Organization (FAO/WHO) determined that the best way to determine protein quality was the Protein Digestibility Corrected Amino Acid Score (PDCAAS). The PDCAAS is based on both the amino acid requirements of humans and their ability to digest it. The highest PDCAAS value comes from casein (milk protein), followed by egg white, soy protein (soybean isolates; a highly refined or purified form of soy protein, which has had most of the non-protein components, fats and carbohydrates removed), whey (another milk protein), beef, soybean (a species of legume native to East Asia), chickpeas, fruits, vegetables, other legumes, cereals and their derivatives, then whole wheat. However, no reference is made to the quality of the milk protein; raw dairy products are much healthier than those that are pasteurized and/or homogenized. Further, many people have allergic responses to dairy products and soy, so they should probably avoid the top four highest protein foods.

Serotonin (or 5-HTP) usually inhibits nerves and is involved in sleep and wakefulness cycles, mood, appetite, and sensitivity. However, it can also be excitatory and is part of the brain's reward system producing feelings of pleasure.

Fermentation vs. Distillation

Fermentation is where all alcohol is created; distillation removes the alcohol from what has been fermented, leaving the distilled alcohol, or spirits.

People who suffer from clinical depression may have too little active serotonin in their synapses (the clefts between where one nerve ends and another begins). They could benefit from enhancing the quality of their serotonin by supplementation. Assessing neurotransmitter function and restoring activity where needed is an important part of improving your brain health. Many people are able to improve their serotonin situation by seeing a functional neurologist or another like-minded alternative healthcare professional (like a naturopath, osteopath, allopath, etc.) who is specially trained to restore the way the human nervous system processes the information it receives from the internal and external environments. Changing the character of the sensory input changes the way the nerve synapses process the signals they relay and the quality of neurotransmitters they contain.

It is said that carbohydrate-based foods such as pasta, starchy vegetables, potatoes, cereals, and breads, which can stimulate serotonin, may cause spikes in blood sugar levels that can contribute to a hypoglycemic response. This means that a person may initially feel good right after eating lots of carbs, but then quickly feels tired. Have you ever seen a family member strewn out on the couch after a big turkey meal (as is so common after Thanksgiving in the U.S.)? They typify the effects of too much tryptophane, which leads to serotonin overload.

If this is you, balancing your blood sugar will increase serotonin's benefits by making your metabolism more efficient. Simple blood tests can help track down the problem, but saliva tests are attracting much attention. They are an easy way to get very reliable information about the causes of hypoglycemia.

Seven Easy Steps to a Clean Brain

Think about this: The functional brain is designed to be tidy not only in the way it processes the incoming and outgoing signals it receives, but also in its processing of nutrients. A healthy brain cannot stand congestion; it requires continued flow and cleansing. A few simple changes can help you keep your brain as healthy and strong as it can be.

Step 1: Eliminate or reduce your consumption of alcohol

Most alcohol has the potential to kill brain cells. It causes brain cells to swell up and burst; it kills them. Alcohol damage can lead to difficulty walking, blurred vision, slurred speech, slowed reaction times, and impaired memory. Clearly, alcohol harms the brain. Some of these functional losses are evident after only one or two drinks and gradually disappear when drinking stops. On the other hand, a person who drinks heavily over a long period of time may have brain deficits that persist well after he or she stops drinking altogether. Exactly how alcohol affects the brain and the likelihood of reversing the impact of heavy drinking on the brain remain hot topics in alcohol research today.

A number of factors influence how and to what extent alcohol affects the brain, including:

- *How much and how often a person drinks;*
- *The age at which (and how long) he or she first began drinking;*
- *The person's age, level of education, gender, genetic background, and family history of alcoholism;*
- *Whether he or she is at risk as a result of prenatal alcohol exposure; and*
- *His or her general health status.*

It is thought that the effects of fermented alcohol (wine and beer) are different than the effect of distilled spirits. However, heavy drinking, no matter what type of alcohol is consumed, may have extensive and far-reaching effects on the brain, ranging from simple "slips" in memory to permanent and debilitating conditions that require lifetime custodial care. And even moderate drinking leads to short–term impairment, as shown by extensive research on the impact of drinking on driving.

Step 2: Stop using tobacco and nicotine products

Anything that contains nicotine will damage the brain's circulation. Nicotine tightens the capillaries, hindering the flow of blood, oxygen, and glucose to the cortical and cerebellar tissues that need them most.

No matter how tobacco is consumed—chewed, snuffed or smoked—the nicotine it contains is a powerful drug, which is the main factor responsible for its dependence-forming properties. According to the American Heart Association, nicotine addiction has historically been one of the hardest addictions to break.

Smoking tobacco makes its nicotine readily available to the lungs, crossing the blood-brain barrier within ten to twenty seconds after inhalation. Its half-life is about two hours. Nicotine can also enter the bloodstream through the mucous membranes that line the mouth (if tobacco is chewed) or nose (if snuff is used), and even through the skin.

Nicotine (including the patch) affects the entire body, acting directly on the heart to change heart rate and blood pressure. It also acts on the nerves that control respiration, altering breathing patterns. In high concentrations, nicotine is deadly; one drop of purified nicotine on the tongue will kill a person. It's so lethal that it has been used as a pesticide for centuries.

> *The blood-brain barrier is a series of tight junctions along the capillaries of the brain that protect the brain tissues from the harmful substances in the circulating blood. If a person has a leaky gut, they have a very high probability of also having a leaky brain.*

So why do people smoke? Nicotine acts in the brain where it can stimulate feelings of pleasure. Its pharmacological and behavioral characteristics are similar to those of heroin and cocaine.

Step 3: Cut the fat

> *Healthy brain foods deliver a steady balance of blood sugars, minimizing the "crash-and-burn" effect.*

Cut hydrogenated and partially hydrogenated fats from your diet. Everything eaten eventually makes its way to the cells that make up tissues, and they compose the organs that participate in life-sustaining processes. This means that hydrogenated fats are terrible for your brain.

Recall the lipid-protein sandwich that makes up the cell's membrane. If eaten, hydrogenated and partially hydrogenated fats get into the cell, changing its structure and function from its original design. These functional tissue changes lead to eventual sickness.

It is a fundamental rule that structure and function are inseparable; structure determines function, and vice versa. A cell's membrane is meant to have a certain type of amino acid and fatty acid structure and anything other than that structure alters its function. Hydrogenated and partially hydrogenated fats present a different structure than that seen in a healthy cell membrane. Altered fats change the signal flow making subsequent nerve impulses respond differently. Nerve signals are designed to flow at a certain pace, and anything that speeds them up or slows them down changes them from their original design.

Consider this: when comparing the short-term effects of nicotine and the long-term effects of these dangerous fats, each leads to circulatory problems, but together they bring about toxicity faster.

Since toxic fats and smoking significantly increase the likelihood of a sick brain, it is a healthy decision to make lifestyle changes that eliminate both dangerous fats and nicotine.

Step 4: Axe the artificial flavorings, colorings, and sweeteners

Artificial ingredients have no place in a natural and healthy diet. Artificial flavorings, artificial sweeteners, or artificial colorings are a brain hazard, proportionally more harmful to children than to adults. Therefore, it behooves parents to keep artificial foods from their children. How can you tell when a food has them? Read labels. "Artificial" and "natural" ingredients are often pseudonyms for "MSG."

Step 5: Avoid simple carbohydrates

Foods that provide quick bursts of energy do so by spiking the blood sugar level, but they are often followed by a crash. These foods are usually carbohydrates made of simple sugars—also known as "simple carbs."

Did you know that there are no essential carbohydrates? As we have seen, there are essential fatty acids and essential amino acids, but carbohydrates are different. While they can supply readily available energy sources, carbohydrates are not essential to the human diet. This means that the human system is able to create any carbohydrate it may need in order to produce energy.

Did you ever notice that the produce in grocery stores usually carries a sticker with several numbers? What do these numbers mean?

Most conventional fruit stickers begin with a "4."

Organic fruit stickers begin with a "9."

Genetically modified organism (GMO) fruit stickers begin with an "8." Beware: There are no big signs that say "GMO." The only evidence that a food contains GMOs is a small sticker that indicates:

"THIS FOOD IS A GMO."

Remember: Any "8" should not be ate, and any "9" is fine.

Managing blood sugar changes is a symphony of organic immersion. The blood sugar balancing mechanisms must all work together to maintain physiological balance. Within the first hour after a meal, the blood sugar normally rises along a physiological course causing the liver and the pancreas to respond. For the first thirty minutes after eating, the liver is very active. It is opening its "gates" to accept blood sugar so it does not rise too quickly. For the next thirty minutes of the first hour, the pancreas is the major worker, secreting insulin that pushes the blood sugar into storage. So, within the first hour after eating, the liver and pancreas work together to manage the increasing blood sugar. In the second hour, the adrenals work to cushion the dropping blood sugar so it comes down slowly and easily.

In the third hours, the adrenals hand off the blood sugar management responsibilities to the thyroid. Hour four sees the increased influence of the gonads—testes and ovaries—then the spleen and thymus in the fifth and sixth hours after eating.

When the body has trouble managing blood sugar, those troubles usually appear within the first two or three hours after eating, indicating liver, pancreas, adrenal, and/or thyroid troubles.

Step 6: Use common sense and choose good "brain foods"

Your brain's energy also comes from the efficient use of blood sugar. Your brain uses at least 20% of all carbohydrates that you ingest, but it prefers it in a specific way—a constant, steady supply, without interruptions or extremes.

Wise food choices are usually consistent with balanced and steady blood sugar levels. Avoid refined sugar products, even the term "natural" (i.e. flavors, colors, and sugars) refined flour products, all drugs, and most types of alcohol. Also, avoid any substance (i.e. Snickers® bars, candies, chips, cakes, cookies, pies, etc.) that you know will give you a ton of initial energy, but cause you to crash-and-burn later.

The Physiological Effects of Blood Sugar

Hours After Eating	Organ
First 30 minutes	Liver
30-60 minutes	Pancreas
2 hours	Adrenal glands
3 hours	Thyroid
4 hours	Gonads
5 hours	Spleen
6 hours	Thymus

Step 7: Improve your mental health

The health of your brain is directly related to your diet. People with emotional or learning troubles often have problems with their blood sugar, and that relates to their diet. Brain health and blood sugar have a direct cause and effect relationship. Most of the time, healthy dietary choices can change your mood and/or reduce its overall intensity.

Summary

A brain that can speak is a peculiar thought, but where do you think those voices in your head come from, anyway? The brain contains the core of who we are and what we believe. It just makes sense to keep your brain free of impurities and to feed it properly. Toxins have a terrible influence on tissues in general, but they are especially damaging to nerves and nerve tissue. Generally, what goes into the mouth eventually shows up in the tissues. Therefore, if health is the goal, thought should be given to what we ingest. If your brain could speak, it would probably say, "I want to be at my best!"

> ## *Eat Right Rule*
>
> *If your food can go bad, it's good for you. If it can't go bad, it's bad for you.*

There is little nutrition on grocery store shelves these days, and any remnant of nutrient has been adulterated by manufacturing, processing, and marketing.

There are plenty of dangers in manufactured foods. They are either calorie-rich-and-nutrient-poor, or they contain additives, dyes, preservatives, trans-fats, gluten, high-fructose corn syrup, MSG—and its many other aliases—and a whole list of other unhealthy items. Not only that, but today's consumers must also be aware of ionizing radiation and microwaves adulterating their food, robbing it of nutritive value while introducing free radicals that make it potentially carcinogenic.

> *All forms of ionizing radiation, including the cobalt-60 and cesium-137 used in food irradiation, are known carcinogens.*

The idea is to obtain all our essential nutrients from food. Food is your best medicine. Consider it your health insurance policy because if you do not eat right, then sickness may be lurking down the road. One of the keys to good health is frequent small live food meals every day, and do not miss a meal. You can either pay now for healthy quality, organic food at the store or pay later in doctor and hospital bills. The choice is yours.

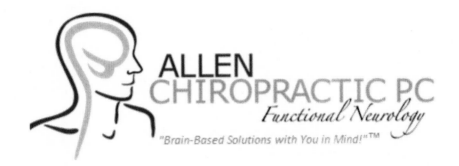

SECTION III

"I LOST THE WORDS!"

CHAPTER SEVEN

IF YOUR BRAIN COULD SPEAK, IT MIGHT SAY...

"I Lost the Words!"

Consider these questions: What is your diet like? Do you only eat when you are hungry? Do you skip meals? Do you skip breakfast? Frequent small meals are very important for a consistent blood sugar level, and that is one of the secrets to helping the brain perform as well as it can.

There is so much nutrition information available these days; what to eat and what to avoid eating. There seems to be a nutritional remedy for just about every ailment imaginable. Everyone, no matter how healthy or fit, wants to be even healthier and fitter.

People who are healthy probably consider that they will always be healthy, and when they are sick, they immediately desire to make the changes that will help them regain their health. While the usual changes may eventually work, they may not always be the answer. One person's nutritional remedy may not be the same for another person with the same problem. For example, Vitamin C may help one person ease his or her cold symptoms, but another person may have plenty of Vitamin C in their system, but they need to avoid dairy or take extra Vitamin A, instead. There are different remedies for different people because no two people's systems are exactly alike.

Left-brain vs. Right-brain

Certain lobes of the human brain specialize in language, with small variations in cortical size from the right side to the left side. These differences may form the basis for lateralization of language to the left hemisphere.

In virtually all right-handers, the left hemisphere processes most language functions. In everybody else (left-handers and those who are ambidextrous), language functions are far more likely to involve the right hemisphere. There is some evidence that lateralization differs in males and females.

There is also evidence that the non-dominant hemisphere is primarily involved in functions that are just one step beyond the essential language functions of relating form to literal meaning. These include determining the emotional state of a speaker from his or her tone of voice, and appreciating humor and metaphor.

Giving Your Brain a Voice

The brain is the most complex part of the human body. It is about the same size as your two fists held side by side, weighs about three pounds and is the seat of your intelligence. It is the interpreter of your senses, initiator of your body movement, and controller of your behavior. Set inside its bony shell and bathed by protective fluid, your brain is the source of all the qualities that define your humanity. In general, the brain is the crown jewel of the human body.

Your brain knows what it needs, and it makes these needs known in both verbal and non-verbal ways. An emotional outburst may indicate the need for Vitamin B complex. Every baby, infant and/or toddler knows how to get its needs met de-

The brain is like a committee of experts. All the parts of the brain work together, but each member has its own special responsibilities.

spite having no language skills. Movements, gestures, and sounds all eventually get the job done. The same is true with the human nervous system.

If your brain could speak, it might say, "I have a lot to say." Although the nervous system does not use words, it communicates through the muscles. The end result of any physiological process is the contraction of a muscle. Your muscles ultimately display your nervous system's condition in a language I call, "neurologese." If we know how to interpret the language of the muscles, we can understand the nervous system's needs.

If your brain is going to express itself, then it must have a voice. Neurochemicals—those unique large molecules that participate in the relaying of a nerve signal from one nerve to another—are that voice.

A Receptor for Every Stimulus

Our bodies are able to perform as a highly organized switchboard, receiving input from the environment by way of our senses, and acting on it—organizing and processing— appropriately. Our senses include the input that comes from the pro-

> *A nerve signal may not be able to jump from one nerve to another if there is inadequate neurotransmitter substance in the synapse.*

cesses of movement and gravity, as well as from our special senses of hearing, seeing, touching, tasting, and feeling. When these systems are all working properly, and the brain is able to correctly interpret the information they send, we refer to this process as sensory integration; the ability to respond to all the senses as though they were one. However, when the sensory input becomes ill-timed, we call that "sensory conflict," or "sensory disconnect."

In general, the neurological chatter that takes place between one nerve and another, or one group of nerves and another group of nerves starts with some sort of receptor stimulation. When the muscle receptors (e.g., those mechanoreceptors for stretch and tension, or hot, cold, light touch, deep touch, taste, hearing, [the sense of smell is unique and will not be discussed here]) become

> *The contour of a receptor molecule determines its functional state. It is much like a lock and key mechanism. If the key fits the lock, things can pass, in this case a nerve signal.*

stimulated in their optimal way, they send nerve signals first to the spinal cord, and then to the brain where the nerve impulses turn into various types of useable data. The incoming muscle stretch and tension data, for example, is processed both in the spinal cord and brain, and then the outgoing signals from the brain make their way back to the cord to regulate reflexive responses in the cord.

Nerve receptors generally respond to one main stimulus, but they can be discharged in other ways, too. For example, receptors for hot and cold are able to perceive hot and cold, but it is all relative to the temperature of the environment. The

> *Excitatory NTs trigger a nerve impulse in the receiving cell, while inhibitory NTs act to prevent further transmission of an impulse.*

ambient temperature influences how the receptors work. Did you ever have fingers so cold that they were numb? How did you warm them? Would you use hot water or cold? When fingers are so cold that they feel numb, even cold water may feel too hot. Further, the hot receptors can be stimulated by friction, rubbing your hands together quickly—the effect of kinetic force between two contrarily-moving solid surfaces.

These receptors that best perceive vision are stimulated by light. When light hits the retina, the visual receptors—which turn light into nerve signals—stimulate the nerves, and their signals eventually reach the brain. Consider this. You could also stimulate your visual receptors by closing your eyes and rubbing them vigorously. You will probably see flashes of light, but is that vision?

> *The gap between neurons is called a synapse. Information flows across the synapse from one neuron to another. The presynaptic ending contains NTs and a few other cell organelles, while the postsynaptic ending contains receptors that receive NTs.*

These two examples show that friction and direct ocular pressure are alternative—but not optimal—ways to discharge the hot and visual receptors, respectively. Further, neither the responses to friction, nor the light sensed by pressure stimulation to the eyes are as meaningful as the perception of hot water or the light that hits the retina providing detail of the outside world. Each receptor has its own primary stimulus for which that receptor is intended.

When your brain needs "stimulating conversation," the most meaningful input you could give it is the input that comes from joint motion. Muscle contraction and the associated joint movement, like the stretch of a tendon or ligament, are the best kind of stimulation for your brain. However, most people answer the brain's request for stimulation by eating or they turn to drugs or medication. Health food stores have a variety of nutrients for your brain, and drug stores are full of over-the-counter medications. The health food stores are full of vitamin, mineral, and protein supplements that can manage blood sugar and nutrient needs. Drugs or medications can produce brain changes, but they always come at a price—drug side effects lead to other problems.

Since the nervous system's primary needs are neurological, nothing short of a neurological remedy will meet these needs. Nutrition may help provide the foundation for brain function, but the benefits are second-best when the brain needs neurological stimulation. And the best neurological remedy is whatever it neurologically takes to stimulate the brain tissue needing help. This could be a specific coupled chiropractic adjustment, or a well-defined type of fast or slow, or complex or simple movement, temperature stimulation to one ear rather than the other, or any other therapy that meets the explicit neurological need.

Amino Acids

Amino acids and the proteins they create excite or calm your nervous system, and nourish it throughout its lifetime. As a general rule of nature, proteins (and their amino acid components) are biologically linked with fatty acids, indicating that nature intends that proteins and fatty acids should work together.

> *While all NTs are NCs, not all NCs are NTs. For example, the nitric oxide molecule is important for transmitting information between cells, but it contains no amino acids; it is a free radical. It may be classified as an NT but it is not included with other NTs because it is not released the same way as an NT.*

Their blending with various vitamins and minerals is essential for developing brains, memory, and learning.

It is estimated that the human body may contain over two million proteins, but nobody really knows how many proteins there are in the human body. The longest known protein, titin, also known as connectin, contains a chain of 26,926 amino acids. Titin is found in muscle and contributes to its passive stiffness.

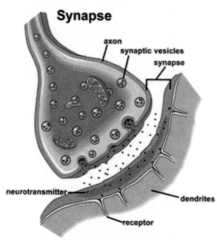

Synapse

The Neuron (Axon), Synaptic Cleft and Neurotransmitters

The twenty-two basic amino acids are the building blocks of life. Like fatty acids that are composed of long molecular chains of various carbon combinations, proteins are made up of long molecular chains of amino acids in a variety of unique combinations. Most neurochemicals (NCs) and neurotransmitters (NTs) are made from amino acids, found in protein-rich foods, and are the building blocks of your brain's neural network. NCs and NTs are special signal-carrying messengers that relay information between different nerve cells or between nerve cells and muscles. They motivate or sedate, focus or frustrate; they shift your mood and change your mind. NTs contain the "words" that tell the status of the human nervous system.

While an electrical signal naturally flows through each neuron, there must be some way to get the signal from the end of one nerve to the beginning of the next. NCs and NTs form a kind of bridge. They are generally made up of amino acids, which are the key components of proteins. Both NCs and NTs relay the nerve signal from nerve to nerve, some passing on the signal and others quieting it.

Neurotransmitters

When a nerve signal comes to the end of a neuron it must either make the transition from that neuron to the next one, or die. If it can jump the synapse, the gap between the neurons, the nerve signal can continue to the end of that neuron and to the end of every neuron thereafter if enough NTs exist. On the other hand, if the synapse has an insufficient quantity of NTs, the nerve signal cannot jump the gap, and the nerve signal just disappears. It can go no further.

Proteins and their Structure

Type of Protein	The Protein's Structure	Significant Bonding
Primary	Linear structure	Covalent (very loosely held)
Secondary	Coiled or spiral shape, or generally twisted, pleated sheet	Hydrogen
Tertiary	A spherical structure; More complicated coils, spirals, twists, or pleats	Generally between amino groups
Quaternary	Interwoven or coiling protein molecules with multiple subunits	Several different bonds exist between the side groups of different chains; van der Waals bonds, hydrogen bonds, ionic bonds, or at times covalent bonds

The delivery end of a neuron is where the excitement happens. These nerve signals are ferried across the synapse from one neuron to a target (receptor) cell on the dendrite of the next neuron, on the backs of NCs and NTs.

NTs are special NCs that are knit together within each neuron from plentiful and simple essential components, such as amino acids, which are readily available from the diet and which require only a small number of biosynthetic steps to convert.

The NCs are found outside the nerve cell while the information-carrying NTs are produced within the nerve cell itself.

NTs are biologically wrapped up into small packets, called vessicles, which are clustered beneath the membrane on the presynaptic (or near-end) side of a two-nerve link. The presence of the nerve signal makes the vessicles pop open and release their contents into the synaptic cleft—the gap between the neurons—forming the bridge. The NTs float through the synaptic cleft, where they act locally to bind to receptors in the membrane on the far (the postsynaptic) side of the synapse. The bridge is complete when the NT molecules fit into special receptors on the receiving end of the next nerve, like a unique key into the exclusive lock that opens the neurological doors to the next neuron so the nerve signal can continue on its way.

Animal protein is generally a complete protein, but even the protein in animal products does not have a perfect amino acid ratio. Animal protein can be as low as 60% usable protein up to about 85% usable protein.

Our brains store long-term memories in these synapse combinations, which are rich in NCs and NTs. But if these nerve signals are lost, they leave the subsequent nerves unstimulated, doing nothing for the rest of the brain and making it more difficult to form memories, if they are able to be formed at all.

What happens if there are too few NCs and/or too few packets of NTs at the ends of the nerves? That is a very important question because it can happen, and that is where many emotional issues such as phobias and depression come from, as does the use of drugs to treat them.

Many people turn to drugs to help their nerves, but while drugs have a particular target, they also have inherent side effects. Your nervous system, however, knows what substances are necessary to do any particular job, and how to do that job, including how to carry a nerve signal.

Goin' on a Road Trip

A nerve's transmission is like going on a road trip. Imagine you and your family are traveling to the next city, and being escorted by a particular person. Not just any person will do, but it has to be a specific person. That person has to be dressed just right, and they have to drive a special car; a very unique car. Only one fixed route will get you there. Does that sound too specific?

The blood-brain barrier has several important functions:
• *Protects the brain from "foreign substances" in the blood that may injure the brain.*
• *Protects the brain from hormones and neurotransmitters in the rest of the body.*
• *Maintains a constant environment for the brain.*

Amino acids face the same dilemma when they jump a synapse or are sent to the brain. Actually, the fact that amino acids are able to make up NCs and NTs at all is an achievement. The groups of cells and neurons that make up the different body tissues all need amino acids to make NCs and NTs, and the tissues obtain these special biochemicals from the blood relatively easily. However, in the brain, the amino acids have to pass through a particular blood-brain barrier that makes their transport a bit trickier. Amino acids compete with each other and with other biochemicals for so many uses in the body that it makes one ponder the exacting wisdom that creates these neurologically essential molecules. More importantly, amino acids must be escorted through the blood-brain barrier by a unique carrier molecule—configured just right—in a certain "vehicle" along a specific route.

What about a Deficiency?

What if the amino acids cannot be converted from their basic components into the necessary NC or NT? Every NC and NT is the result of a specific metabolic pathway that involves certain essential components without which that pathway cannot be completed. If the essential components that knit the NC or NT together in the synapse are unavailable where they are needed, one might use a drug or medication to simulate the NC's or the NT's natural presence, but that is quite possibly one of the least appropriate ways to make the synapse work. Treating neurological problems with pharmaceuticals has a high probability of inviting side effects. Giving a drug to make an NC and/or an NT is not the same as providing an environment that enables your body to make its own biochemicals.

A certain drug might work initially, but their effect very often wears off over time leading to the need for another, more powerful drug in its place. Drug doses must often be modified and sensitivities can develop. Not everyone can take the same drug for the same problem, which means that some people must change to a different drug and hope for the same benefit.

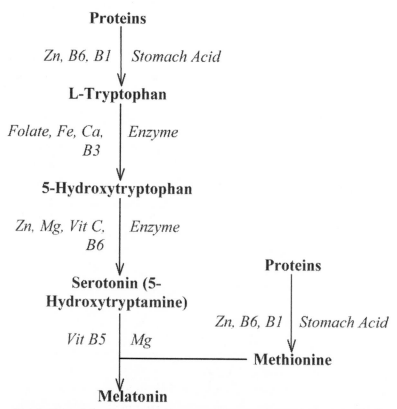

Proteins

Zn, B6. B1 | Stomach Acid

L-Tryptophan

Folate, Fe, Ca, B3 | Enzyme

5-Hydroxytryptophan

Zn, Mg, Vit C, B6 | Enzyme

Proteins

Serotonin (5-Hydroxytryptamine)

Zn, B6, B1 | Stomach Acid

Vit B5 | Mg

Methionine

Melatonin

Metabolism of the Neurochemical Melatonin from Another Neurochemical Methionine, via Proteins with Associated Neurotransmitters Tryptophan and Serotonin, and Key Essential Components (Zn=Zinc; Fe=Iron; Ca=Calcium; Mg=Magnesium)

Further, drugs have to be broken down like everything else in the body. This means that a tissue's essential components that could have been used for other needs must be siphoned off to another locale to metabolize the drugs that might not have needed to be there in the first place. Slowly but surely the tissues adapt to these changing dynamics, eventually compromising the way the tissues express themselves; they develop a "normal" that is different from their original intent. When the essential components for repair are not available, it can lead to an NC or an NT deficiency, which makes the system work in a way contrary to its optimal performance. Pathology is the result. All these pharmaceutical effects ultimately display themselves in the way the muscles work, and that compromises structural stability. If your brain could speak, it might say, "Excuse me. I do not need drugs. I would rather do it myself!"

Some Common NTs

The only direct action of an NT is to activate a receptor. Therefore, the usefulness of an NT system depends on the connections of the neurons that use the NT, and the chemical properties of the receptors to which the NT binds. In general, NTs influence the performance of *the next neuron* in a series. They are also found at the axon endings of motor neurons, where they stimulate the muscle fibers. NTs and their close relatives—the NCs—are also produced by glands such as the pituitary and the adrenal glands. Some NTs have an excitatory affect and others have an inhibitory affect.

Excitatory NTs

Glutamate

Most fast excitatory synapses in the brain and spinal cord—as much as half of all neurons in the brain—are associated with the NT, glutamate, an excitatory relative of GABA. Glutamate is the most common neurotransmitter in the central nervous system and is especially important with regards to memory. Once glutamate bursts into the synapse, its presence unlocks the receptors at the receiving end of the adjacent neuron, and then it lingers in the synapse to encour-

> *Inflammation is not the same as infection. Without inflammation, wounds or infections could not heal. However, because chronic inflammation can lead to a host of other immune conditions, inflammation is closely regulated by the body.*

age other nerve signals along their course. However, glutamate is actually toxic to neurons. While it excites a subsequent neuron and spurs the signal on to its ultimate destination, too much glutamate can actually kill neurons. Sometimes brain damage or a stroke will lead to an excessive amount of glutamate, ultimately killing more brain cells than the original trauma. Additionally, too little glutamate can cause tiredness and poor brain activity, but too much may make you feel anxious and depressed, or lead to seizures, psychological and immunological symptoms.

Acetylcholine

"To excite or inhibit, that is the question." The effects of NTs often depend on where in the body they are sent to work. Acetylcholine works in the peripheral nervous system to excite the nerve-muscle junction to cause contraction of skeletal muscle, but when it works in the heart, it inhibits the contraction of heart muscle. Further, when considering its effects on the central nervous system, acetylcholine has an overall anti-excitatory effect. A deficiency of acetylcholine can cause difficulty remembering common facts about other people, like names, faces, birthdays, or telephone numbers. A deficiency can also cause disorientation, isolation, despair, lack of creativity and imagination, as well as difficulty remembering lists, directions, or instructions. There are no known issues with having too much acetylcholine.

Excitatory Neurotransmitters: Their Functions and Levels

Neurotransmitter Key: NT = Neurotransmitter; * = Regulate Mood † = Neuromuscular; ‡ = Neuromodulator	Functions	Low levels can cause...	High levels can cause...
Glutamate (Glu)	The primary excitatory NT, necessary for learning and memory	Tiredness and poor brain activity	Anxiety, low mood, seizures, psychological and immunological symptoms
Acetylcholine (ACh)†‡	Related to autonomic regulation; main NT in the spinal cord	Forgetfulness, hard to find the right words, low libido, slow or confused thinking, weakened memory, disorientation, and decreased creativity	No known clinical symptoms to date
Aspartic Acid (Asp)	Vital for energy and brain function	Tiredness and low mood	Seizures and anxiety
Epinephrine (Epi)	AKA adrenaline; vital for motivation, energy, and mental focus	Fatigue, lack of focus, difficult losing weight	Sleep difficulties, anxiety, and attention issues
Norepinephrine (Nor)*	Mental focus and emotional stability	Lack of: energy, focus, motivation; and low mood	Anxiety, stress, and high blood pressure; hyperactivity

(Table continued from page 229)

Neurotransmitter Key: *NT = Neurotransmitter;* ** = Regulate Mood* *† = Neuromuscular;* *‡ = Neuromodulator*	Functions	Low levels can cause...	High levels can cause...
Dopamine (Dop)*‡	Feelings of pleasure and satisfaction, muscle control and function	Addictions and cravings	Poor intestinal function, develop-mental delay, and attention issues
PEA	Important for focus and con-centration	Inattentiveness, unclear think-ing, and depres-sion	"Racing mind," sleep dif-ficulties, anxiety, and schizo-phrenia
Histamine (His)‡	The pacemaker; controls energy, motivation, and sleep-wake cycles	Feeling tired	Allergic responses and sleep difficulties

Epinephrine

Epinephrine is another excitatory NT, also known as adrenaline. It increases heart rate, constricts blood vessels, dilates air passages, and participates in the fight-or-flight response. It is important for motivation, energy, and mental focus. Too little of it can be a reason for fatigue, difficulty focusing, and making it hard to lose weight. Too much of it can lead to sleep difficulties, anxiety, and attention issues.

Norepinephrine

As a stress hormone, norepineph-rine affects parts of the brain, such as the amygdala, where attention and responses are controlled. Stress tends to deplete our store of adrenalin—epinephrine and norepinephrine—while exercise tends to increase our stores. Together with epinephrine, norepinephrine also underlies the fight-or-flight response, directly increasing heart rate, triggering the release of glucose from energy stores, and increasing blood flow to skeletal muscle. Norepineph-rine increases the brain's oxygen supply, and it can suppress neurological inflammation when released by certain parts of the brain. An excess of norepinephrine can lead to nervousness, tension, hyperactivity, and high blood pressure, while a deficiency can cause a lack of energy, focus and motivation, and a compromised mood.

> *Certain drugs can damage the brain's cognitive abilities, especially in elderly patients.*
>
> *Mitochondria are the inevitable target of statin drugs—like the drug Crestor®—leaving the mitochondria fully exposed to the mutagenic effect of free radicals. However, current literature offers conflicting data with regard to the effects of statins on memory loss.*

Dopamine

Dopamine—a close relative to epinephrine and norepinephrine—comes from several different parts of, and has many effects on, the brain. It acts as a stimulant to the pleasure center of the brain, increasing the heart rate and blood pressure; and it plays important roles in behavior and cognition, voluntary movement, motivation, punishment and reward, inhibition of prolactin production (involved in lactation and sexual gratification), sleep, mood, the ability to pay attention, working memory, and learning. Dopamine is strongly associated with reward mechanisms in the brain. If it feels good, dopamine neurons are probably involved! A dopamine deficiency can create addictions and cravings, while an excess can cause poor intestinal function, developmental delay, and attention issues.

PEA

PEA (short for beta-phenylethyl-amine) is an excitatory neurotrans-mitter normally synthesized in the brain from the amino acid phenyl-alanine. It is important for good focus and concentration. PEA acts as an excitatory neurotransmitter and supersensitizes nerve signals in fa-

> *A brain pacemaker emits periodic signals that disrupt other signals that are out of time with those that are of greater importance, in order to eliminate symptoms.*

vor of glutamate activity and neurotransmitter firing. This promotes energy and elevates mood while it inhibits the re-uptake of dopa-mine and norepinephrine, allowing them to linger in the synapse a bit longer in order to prolong their effect. PEA is a powerful weapon in the fight against aging. It is a research-proven mood-brightener that can quickly boost a depressive mood of sadness, hopelessness, discouragement, and feeling "down in the dumps." It increases the effects of dopamine (for wellbeing and feeling pleasure), norepi-nephrine (the brain's stimulant for wakefulness and higher perfor-mance), acetylcholine (for improving memory and mental activity), and serotonin (for better mood emotion and impulse control).

PEA is a highly-concentrated neurotransmitter in the brain's emo-tional center (the limbic system) that increases motivation, physical drive, feelings, and social activity. Too little PEA can indicate de-pression, difficulty paying attention or thinking clearly, and psycho-pathic symptoms. Too much PEA is an indicator of a biochemical abnormality called phenylketonuria (PKU), which is the absence of the enzyme that helps to synthesize phenylalanine into tyrosine. Too much PEA has been found in patients with a "racing mind," sleep problems, anxiety, and schizophrenia. Also, supplementation that manipulates PEA can help increase focus and attention.

Histamine

Histamine is an excitatory neurotransmitter involved in a wide array of biological actions, including the sleep-wake cycle and inflamma-tory response, which is commonly associated with the exposure to an allergen.

Interestingly, histamine-containing neurons have been found to have a pacemaker function within the brain, showing a relationship with brain activity levels and displaying distinct day-night rhythms. These neurons provide the stimulation that maintains or modulates activity in many other regions of the brain. Too little histamine can lead to tiredness, while too much can cause allergic responses and sleep difficulties.

Inhibitory NTs

GABA

GABA (gamma amino butyric acid) is the chief inhibitory neurotransmitter—meaning that when it finds its way to its receptor sites, it blocks the tendency of that neuron to fire. It is a biochemical found naturally in the body that works in the brain to transmit nerve impulses that mod-

> *Most NTs are either rapidly removed, or recycled and stored for later use. Appropriate NTs should linger and encourage persistence of a nerve's signal.*

ify neuronal excitability throughout the whole nervous system. It inhibits nerve transmission in the brain, calming nervous activity. In humans, GABA is also directly responsible for the regulation of muscle tone. Too little GABA can cause symptoms of hyperactivity, anxiety, panic attacks, seizure disorders, and sleep difficulties. GABA's side effects are mild and uncommon, however, some indications of too much GABA may be wheezing, increased respiratory rate, tachycardia, fidgetiness, anxiety, vomiting, nausea, flushing, and/or tingling in the hands and other parts of the body.

Glycine

> *Gut problems are characteristically related to behavior and learning.*

Glycine is an inhibitory neurotransmitter of the central nervous system, highly concentrated in the spinal cord, brainstem, and retina. Research has shown that this amino acid can help inhibit the neurotransmitters that cause seizure activity, hyperactivity, and manic (bipolar) depression. While there is no real evidence of problems related to too little glycine, too much glycine may be related to anxiousness, low mood, nausea and vomiting, upper digestive tract discomfort, mild drowsiness, and stress-related disorders. Studies have shown that glycine also helps improve memory retrieval loss in those that suffer from a wide variety of sleep-depriving conditions, including schizophrenia, Parkinson's disease, Huntington's disease, jet lag, and overwork.

Taurine

Taurine is said to be conditionally essential: most people do not need to obtain it from dietary sources, as the human body can make taurine on its own, however, it may need supplementation under certain circumstances, such as formula-fed infants or people undergoing IV feedings. Taurine may have several different roles in the human body.

It plays a role in the stimulation of photoreceptors in the function of the retina of the eye, blood platelet activity, sperm motility, insulin activity, regulation of the nervous system, and the formation of bile. It is important for proper heart function, healthy sleep, and promoting calmness. Too little taurine can cause severe symptoms of hyperactivity, anxiousness, and sleep difficulties. Little is known about the effects of too much of heavy or long-term use of taurine. Because the heart is the storage unit for the majority of taurine in the body, an excess amount of taurine over long periods may be related to the developing of heart disease. Some reports indicate that taurine might make a bipolar disorder worse, so play it safe and avoid too much taurine!

Serotonin

Serotonin, sometimes referred to as the happiness hormone, is an inhibitory neurotransmitter that regulates many functions, including mood, appetite, sensory perception, as well as gastrointestinal activity, heart rate, and breathing. However, while a little bit is good, a lot is not better. The "Serotonin syndrome" is the name for a condition when the body has too much serotonin. It can cause restlessness, hallucinations, loss of coordination, fast heartbeat, rapid changes in blood pressure, increased body temperature, overactive reflexes, nausea, vomiting, and diarrhea. Too little serotonin has been shown to lead to depression, problems with anger control, obsessive-compulsive disorder, and suicide. It can also lead to an increased appetite for carbohydrates (starchy foods) and may affect sleep patterns, which are also associated with depression and other emotional disorders. Too little serotonin has also been tied to migraines, irritable bowel syndrome, and fibromyalgia.

Inhibitory Neurotransmitters: Their Functions and Levels

Neurotransmitter Key: NT = Neurotransmitter; * = Regulate Mood; ‡= Neuromodulator	Functions	Low levels can cause...	High levels can cause...
GABA*	Primary inhibitory NT; necessary to feel calm and relaxed	Severe hyperactivity, anxiousness, and sleep difficulties	Wheezing, tingling hands and other body parts, anxiety, vomiting, nausea, flushing, increased respiratory rate, tachycardia, and fidgetiness
Glycine (Gly)	Much like GABA; helps calm and relax the body	No known clinical symptoms to date	Anxiousness, low mood, and stress-related disorders
Taurine (Tau)	Important for proper heart function, healthy sleep, and promoting calmness	Severe hyperactivity, anxiousness, and sleep difficulties	Little is known about heavy or long-term use; it might make bipolar disorder worse

(Table Continued from Page 235)

Neurotransmitter Key: NT = Neurotransmitter; * = Regulate Mood; ‡= Neuromodulator	Functions	Low levels can cause...	High levels can cause...
Serotonin (Ser)*‡	Resolution of mood, sleep, and appetite	Depression, sleep difficulties, hot flashes, anger control problems, headache, uncontrolled appetite, obsessive-compulsive disorder, and suicide	Serotonin syndrome; rapid blood pressure changes, coordination loss, nausea, vomiting, & diarrhea, hyperactive reflexes, restlessness, tachycardia, hallucinations, and elevated body temperature

More about Neurotransmitters

Most NTs become recycled by local enzymes, which demands a constant input of the essential components for repair—like amino acids, micronutrients, vitamins, and minerals—to rebuild them again. This also requires the fuel (i.e., glucose and oxygen) necessary for function, and the antioxidants necessary for protection. If any one or a combination of these essential components for repair is missing, it can compromise the way the NT works, producing erroneous issues of perception, behavior, cognition, and mood.

Neurological Exercise

Just like the rest of your body, your nervous system needs exercise. We all think of exercise as doing cardio, lifting weights, Pilates, yoga, running, etc. These exercises all work the muscles, lungs, and

---

The Five Most Common Prescriptions (2009)

The most popular (#1) prescription drug in the United States is hydrocodone with acetaminophen—the active ingredient in Tylenol®; a painkiller—sold under the name Vicodin®. There were 128.2 million prescriptions in 2009 at a cost of about $12 a month.

#2: There were 83 million prescriptions for the most widely prescribed cholesterol drug, Simvastatin® (Zocor®).

#3: High blood pressure is most often treated with the ACE inhibitor, Lisinopril® (Prinivil® and Zestril®), with 81.3 million prescriptions.

#4: 66 million prescriptions for Levothyroxine® sodium (thyroid disorders), because bodies do not produce enough of their own thyroid hormone.

#5: Azithromycin® (an antibiotic), was prescribed 53.8 million times because of its convenient dosing and relatively benign side effects.

Rounding out the next ten most popular medications, are those for diabetes, high cholesterol, five for high blood pressure (with and without angina), an antibiotic, one for heartburn, and one for anxiety.

Source: Forbes.com

---

heart to keep them strong. Neurological exercise is no different. The exercise signals from muscle and organ stimulation start in the periphery and travel to the brain. These exercise signals run through the nerves, making them perform at a higher rate than they would when the body is inactive.

When muscles work hard, their signals make everything along their neurological path perform at a higher rate. In a *perfect* world, all the incoming signals work according to their original design. Stimulation generates signals that pass to the spinal cord creating a flurry of NT display that enhances the stimulation according to their original design. However, in the *real* world, systems often work other than how they should, and pathways tend to break down. When a peripheral stimulation exceeds a pathway's functional capacity—i.e., when the stimulus exceeds the available ingredients for response—that system's inner workings get interrupted with resulting dysfunction.

Good and Bad Plasticity

Previously, we discussed how plasticity can be either helpful or harmful. *Euplasticity*—like *eu*stress—is the reinforcement that helps build the nervous system according to its original design. Euplasticity works in conjunction with the nervous system's fundamental plan that each aspect of the nervous system works to the benefit of every other aspect. Conversely, dysplasticity—plasticity

---

Meet Daniel, 23 years old, college student

It is possible to develop a specific neurotransmitter deficiency should the essential components for its production be unavailable. Each specific neurotransmitter requires its own unique vitamin, mineral, and/or amino acid combinations that enable the cascade of steps that bring about its assembly. Should any one or a blend of these factors be missing, the cascade could quite possibly take an unexpected path, creating a completely different substance.

Reconsider the hose and water analogy from earlier. The water flow of each hose can only occur if sufficient stimulus and nutrients are present. Should the proprioceptive stimulus wane, then so does the water's flow through that hose. Likewise, should there be insufficient nutrients to build the neurotransmitters that would conduct the proprioceptive signal, then the signal would also wane.

Daniel—23 years old—complained of anxiety, nausea, vomiting, digestive issues, depression, sleep difficulties, and emotional restlessness. His examination revealed a specific vitamin complex deficiency that impacted his ability to make a certain neurotransmitter. He often ate on the run and under stress, his foods were poor in substance and lacked life, and his sleep cycles were interrupted. He would go to bed after midnight but wake soon afterwards, staying awake sometimes for an hour or two, falling to sleep again and sleeping late into the morning. Once his habits were changed and his nutrient deficiency was addressed, Daniel's symptoms abated and he felt like a new person almost immediately.

---

that conflicts with the original neurological design—tends toward pathology. Dysplastic nerve signals still generate NTs, but by virtue of their dysfunctional nature, dysplasticity produces more neurological hindrance than reinforcement, therefore dysplasticity suppresses the type of nerve signal that is needed in order to make the nervous system work optimally.

Long term dysplasticity eventually makes people realize something is wrong; they just do not feel right. They may experience pain because joint dysfunction eventually leads to pain. Pain is the primary reason people go to the doctor. They describe various aches and pains, and a generalized sense that their body is going downhill and they turn to their doctor for a solution. Whereas people used to be able to tolerate their symptoms or take an over-the-counter medication for temporary relief, that tactic no longer works. Following an examination the patient is often told that there is nothing drastically wrong, but perhaps they should take something to help their pain, elevated cholesterol, high blood pressure, thyroid, blood sugar imbalance, or anxiety to help them feel better, so they take a drug. Do not let this happen to you! Call a functional neurologist or other alternative healthcare professional who understands these issues and get the *real* help you need.

Muscle Input and Brain Outflow

It is a neurological fact that joint motion knocks out pain. Muscles move joints, joints do not move muscles. A functional joint is the result of muscles that work with a balanced give-and-take. When one muscle contracts, the muscle that does the opposite function must relax. That balanced muscle input generates a steady and stable neurological outflow that is important for a healthy and pain-free nervous system.

Of all the outgoing signals from the brain, 90% relate to organ function and only 10% goes to muscles. That makes it much more important to understand organ function than it is to simply exercise muscles.

What are the benefits of neurological exercise when drugs do for the nervous system what the nervous system should be doing for itself? Drugs—those manufactured agents that cause a pharmacological reaction rather than allowing the body to respond physiologically—are designed to change the way receptors work. They block some receptors and stimulate others to demand a particular response

> *This is a very important point: receptors need the right lock and key combination in order to ignite neurological signals.*

despite what the nervous system might want to display. However, pathways that are naturally stimulated according to their original design will in fact produce the specific NT and use it where it is needed.

The All-or-None Theory

A nerve either sends its signal or it is quiet, there is no middle ground; there is no "maybe" zone. This is called the "all-or-none theory." Each receptor must receive an adequate and appropriate stimulation before their nerve can send its signal. That stimulus depends on timing and intensity. If the stimulus is inadequate to generate a nerve signal, or if the NT configuration is impotent, that nerve cannot fire. However, if the stimulus reaches the neurological threshold, and if the NT is built with the right ingredients, that nerve will conduct its signal to the very end. If your brain could speak, it might say, "I want everything or nothing at all!"

One Good Nerve Influences Another

> $A \rightarrow B$
>
> *If C $\rightarrow$ A, then no B*
>
> *C $\rightarrow$ D $\rightarrow$ therefore,*
> *stimulus continues.*

There are many types of synapses, but in general, one nerve excites another, and the signal continues to its destination (A to B, in the diagram, to the left). However, some nerves are designed to cause inhibition, but they, too, must be excited in order for them to do their job of inhibiting the next nerve in the sequence (C to A, in the diagram). Further, if an inhibitory nerve synapses on another inhibitory nerve (considering that D was an inhibitory nerve), the first inhibitory nerve keeps the second inhibitory nerve from inhibiting, the net result being a lack of inhibition, therefore, allowing other nerves upon which D might synapse to continue their journeys.

Synthesis of Thyroid Hormones

The brain's primary need is a neurological stimulus that produces the desired NT. That is, a stimulation that sends the most dynamic signal to the area needing more NTs. Knowing how to do that requires more than a basic understanding of neurology, and that is exactly what we do at **Allen Chiropractic, PC**—and other functional neurologists do, also—when someone's brain needs help. Because of our highly specialized neurology training, we have a unique understanding about how to enable the human nervous system to work according to its optimal design.

The Metabolism of NTs

An example: dopamine and norepinephrine are two NTs that may be deficient in some children. To make these two NTs, there must be adequate supplies of the basic amino acids, also Vitamin B6, and iron in the brain. If a child—or even an adult—does not ingest and properly absorb these nutrients—if the essential components for their production are not available in the

> *If phenylalanine is deficient in the diet, then tyrosine must be supplemented.*

diet—he or she will not have what it takes to make enough dopamine and/or norepinephrine. That can lead to behavioral and emotional troubles.

Imagine that the predictable metabolic pathway that processes one NT into another is like a series of "rivers" running through the body. Do not let "Like a River" diagram below disturb you. Recognize the transition of one NT to another. One "molecule" flows to another, then on into a third, and so forth. The river flows smoothly when the essential components—vitamins, minerals, oxygen, sugar, etc.—are available. That is how the metabolism of one substance predictably becomes another every time in the human system.

Now consider "the river" diagram again. It is the cascade of just one non-essential amino acid, tyrosine; it does not have to be obtained directly through the diet. Tyrosine is the product of the breakdown of the amino acid phenylalanine in the liver (look closely; the only difference between tyrosine and phenylalanine is the "HO-" on the tyrosine), and is found in the nerve cells of the brain. With the help of its essential components—enzymes, folic acid, niacin (Vitamin B3), and iron—tyrosine breaks down to DOPA (by adding another "HO-" to the ring). Then, with the help of Vitamin B6, DOPA

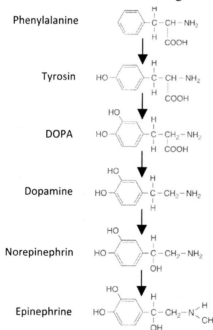

Phenylalanine

Tyrosin

DOPA

Dopamine

Norepinephrin

Epinephrine

Like a River: the Metabolic Pathways of Phenylalanine to Epinephrine

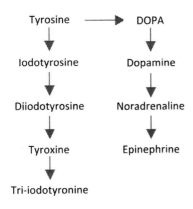

Metabolism of Tyrosine to DOPA and Thyroid Hormones, Dopamine, Noradrenaline and Adrenaline

changes into the dopamine family of hormones (by removing the "-COOH"). Dopamines are synthesized in the adrenal medulla and central nervous system, and they regulate central and peripheral nervous system activity by means of hormones. These NTs include norepinephrine (by adding an oxygen atom) and epinephrine (by removing an "H" and adding a "-CH3"). Easy!

The diagram ("Synthesis of Thyroid Hormones", page 241) above shows that tyrosine is also the source of the thyroid hormones thyroxin (T4) and triiodothyronine (T3), as well as dopamine, noradrenaline and adrenaline.

To cascade from one NT into another requires a full complement of essential components to make the process flow. When those cofactors are not available, it is as if those rivers get dammed up and the waters above the dam swell and those below the dam shrivel. That is what makes one NT linger in a synapse too long while another can be lacking. Further, substituting one atom for another can mean the difference between a metabolic pathway taking one course, as opposed to it taking another metabolic pathway and producing a molecule that is potentially harmful rather than the one that is needed.

As the above examples illustrate, amino acids alone will not make new NTs, neither do single vitamins or minerals. A host of dietary cofactors are critical in order to make the proper brain biochemicals and structures that support optimal mood, cognition, and behavior. However, despite the available nutrients, the key is getting the right kind of stimulation to the nerve to cause the making of the necessary NTs. The nerves must be stimulated according to the human system's original design so that the right NT will be produced to do its job on the following nerve.

Despite all this discussion about nutrients, the key to a healthy brain lies in the quality of incoming nerve signals that arise from the receptors in the muscles and joints. Without that stimulation—without the nerve signals coming along the nerves in the first place—there would be no need for these NTs. Coupled chiropractic adjustments will keep these incoming nerve signals timed properly.

Brain Function: A Matter of Timing

The terms "strong" and "weak" are commonly used in place of the more formal terms "facilitated" and "inhibited," respectively.

If your car's engine is mistimed, it runs rough; and an orchestra that is out of sync sounds cacophonous. Your brain's ability to process information is no different. Your brain's timing is managed by NTs, specifically acetylcholine; they synchronize your brain.

A neuro-typical brain processes a thought in about 320 milliseconds (1/3 of a second). When, eventually, that function slows down by just 25% to 400 milliseconds, logical processes crash, endangering the factors for proper brain function, leading to reduced performance. What was originally designed according to one set of limits adjusts itself to another set of factors that become the new normal, but they are not properly timed for the system as a whole.

People ask me how they can tell if their brain function is slowing down. The truth is that people cannot perceive what they cannot recognize. That is, people cannot tell how their own brains are working because a brain that has troubles cannot sense that it is having trouble. People acclimate to dysfunction, and since they are not aware that they are having trouble, that breakdown is perceived as the "new" normal.

Whether your doctor tests your muscles or not, your muscles speak your brain's level of health. Muscle testing is a wonderful window into your brain's functional capacity because your muscle's level of performance always comes down to the timing of your spinal cord.

Discovering a brain's functional character requires a skilled doctor who knows what to look for and what to do about fixing timing problems when they are found. This is a functional neurologist's forté. This is what we do.

FACT: The average person loses 7-10 milliseconds (2-3%) of brain speed every decade starting at about the age of forty. That loss may not seem like much, but many learning disabilities, psychological problems, and other seemingly unrelated health problems like memory loss or dementias can be linked to slower brain speeds, and 10 milliseconds is a lot when it comes to your brain's timing. A mistimed brain is just one of hundreds of health issues related to brain chemistry.

The same idea is true for manual muscle testing. When a strong muscle that is expected to be strong actually becomes weak (or an expected weak muscle becomes strong), it is theoretically because the spinal cord and brain are unable to update the incoming neurological information fast enough. After treatment, when that previously unexpectedly weak muscle becomes strong again,

> *Our genetics express themselves relative to the quantity of our inflammation. The greater the inflammation, the quicker our genetics will express themselves. If we are genetically predisposed to a certain illness or disease, the faster it will manifest itself.*

(as would be anticipated) there is a very high probability that indicates that the timing between that particular muscle and the cord and brain is back in sync. It is as if the link between the muscle and brain had been speaking different languages; they lost the words that would keep them working together.

The brain is an extremely metabolically active organ. Exercising the brain makes it a very hungry and fussy eater. Recall that the brain's greatest needs are functional nerve signals, oxygen, glucose, blood, and the right food—with all the natural neurochemical cofactors that these foods contain. These factors enhance the brain's mental capabilities and help it concentrate. Supplying the brain with the essential components it needs to work at its highest level helps tune its sensory and motor skills, and keeps it motivated. A motivated brain magnifies one's memory, speeds one's reaction times, diffuses one's stress, and even prevents one's brain from aging. Secondary to neurological stimulation, the brain's biochemical needs cannot be ignored.

Keys to a Healthy Brain

✓ Your nervous system's primary function is to stimulate your brain, and nothing does that better than the sweet experience of nerves that work according to their original design. Dynamically balanced, inflammation-free, coupled motion is the key to a healthy brain.

> *One of the most important keys to a focused brain during the day is to eat a healthy breakfast; high protein is usually best.*

✓ While the right foods are essential for proper brain function, of all the meals in a day, breakfast is the most important meal. The brain is best fueled by a steady supply of glucose, and many studies have shown that skipping breakfast reduces daily academic and work-related performance.

✓ Another one of the first nutrition rules I learned was to eat breakfast like a king or queen, lunch like a prince or princess, and dinner like a pauper. It made a lot of sense to me so I tried it. To my surprise, I was able to pay closer attention throughout my day and had better sleep when I ate a good breakfast and tapered off my caloric intake through the day.

> *Most people have some level of dehydration; they drink too little water. Be sure to prepare your water each morning and drink all of it by the end of your day. If you leave it to thirst, you probably will maintain your dehydration.*

The best breakfasts are higher in protein and balanced with essential fatty acids, minerals, and greens. Around my house, breakfast is a protein drink made with a high quality protein and organic green powder, all added to a whole foods detoxifier, and then blended in a dairy-free almond, rice, or grain milk with a few ice cubes; often I just use water, instead. It is the highlight of the day for me and my kids. It promotes fat loss, helps maintain muscle mass, promotes vitality and energy, naturally normalizes the appetite, and "it sticks to the ribs!"

✓ Among other ideas, a smart choice for lunch is an omelette and also a salad made with carrots, beets, tomatoes, and other healthy vegetables. Avoid iceberg lettuce; it has no nutrient value. Get lettuce that has lots of color—like organic kale, romaine, bib, or organic field greens, for example—and blend them together for the greatest benefit. Healthy vegetables are packed full of antioxidants, including beta-carotene, and Vitamins A, B, C, and E, and lots of minerals that help heal the aging brain, keeping it in tip-top condition by mopping up the damaging free radicals.

To convert pounds to kilograms, divide your weight in pounds by 2.2. Sometimes that is too much math, so approximate it by dividing by 2. That puts you in the ballpark, and that is good.

Another protein drink might also be a good lunch idea. Put some protein powder in a shaker cup and bring along water or your favorite non-dairy liquid. This is what I often do during a busy day at work. It is easy to make, you can *spend your time drinking it slowly*, and the cleanup is easy. A protein drink at lunch is eating like a prince (or princess). Besides, it maintains the blood sugar within optimal limits, and that helps brain power.

✓ Dinner should be high in protein, a balanced amount and healthy source of fatty acids, and complex carbohydrates, but small in quantity, and not eaten too late.

✓ One additional healthy rule: Always eat your food slowly and chew until all solids are liquid.

✓ Make sure you avoid anything white—white breads, white sugars, white flours. Especially avoid highly processed goodies like cakes, pastries, cookies, biscuits—all of which often contain trans-fatty acids—and simple carbohydrates. They are *all* junk foods.

✓ Another general rule that stayed with me is to eat a diet of frequent small meals that are high in protein, low in (simple) carbohydrates, and plenty of fresh raw fruits and vegetables, seeds, nuts, and whole grains; make your diet at least 85% raw and include plenty of healthy oils.

✓ Most people should drink 1.5 to 2 liters of water a day (or you can drink one ounce of water per kilogram of body weight) to keep the brain and other tissues well hydrated.

✓ Oxygenate your brain with aerobic exercise within your personal boundaries (see the 180 Formula, page 146).

When you put these rules into practice, healthy things happen. Eating properly helps provide a constant supply of essential nutrients that can repair tissues and maintain optimal blood sugar levels while avoiding the non-foods that cause detriment and that helps your brain, too. When your brain gets a constant supply of high-grade nutrients while maintaining an appropriate blood sugar level, with plenty of oxygen, it hums along smoothly. My staff often wonders how I can keep going for so long without having to stop to take a break. My diet makes the difference.

A Comment about Protein Consumption

> *Some amino acids are necessary in the diet for children, but not for adults. Those needed only in the diets of children are sometimes called "semi essential."*

Nutrition is a vital part of health. When it comes to food, besides essential fatty acids and the types of carbohydrates they consume, I regularly ask patients about their protein intake. A sufficient daily protein intake is an absolute requirement for overall health, building muscle, maintaining muscle while losing fat, keeping you full and satisfied, and helping you naturally burn more calories each day.

Proteins are one of the most essential components a person can eat, yet there is a lot of controversy surrounding the subject of protein requirements. Few patients understand their daily protein need, and which forms are best.

The primary structure of each protein molecule is the basis of its identity with various amino acids being arranged in different combinations; each combination is as unique as its name. Modification of only one amino acid sequence creates a different protein. Any change of the protein structure is relevant if it alters its biological activity. These structure changes are modifications in the composition of the molecule and such composition determines all other structures of the protein and their uses, as in the cellular membrane.

Complementary Proteins

Combining incomplete sources of vegetable protein provides you with the full complement of essential amino acids. (Choose one from each list; dairy is also allowed)		
Legumes	**Grains**	**Nuts & Seeds**
Black-eyed peas	Rye	Almonds
Chickpeas	Bulgur	Peanuts
Green peas	Couscous	Sunflower
Kidney beans	Oats	Cashews
Lentils	Corn	Sesame
Lima beans	Rice	Walnuts
White beans	Sesame seeds	Pumpkin
Dried peas	Barley	Other nuts
(Sprouted) soy products	Buckwheat	Other seeds

Protein Sources

The majority of my patients tell me that they eat plenty of protein; that they eat some protein source with every meal in the form of beef, poultry, fish, cheese, and eggs; they even put dairy in the list. Sometimes people tell me that they obtain their proteins from beans. But setting environment, hormone and antibiotic use issues aside, while these may all be good sources of protein, they are usually cooked. Isn't that right? When was the last time you ate raw beef, poultry or fish. (Well, where I come from, they call raw fish "bait"!) Some people are comfortable eating raw eggs. That is an individual choice.

All human proteins contain only twenty different amino acids in endless variations. A proper ratio of essential amino acids is necessary for building protein, which is vital to constructing and supporting your tissues, from your cells to your nerves, and from your bones to your muscles. Animal protein, such as meat, poultry, eggs, fish, milk, and cheese provide all of the essential amino acids, but their ratio is unlike human protein.

Better and Lesser Protein Sources

Better Protein Source	Lesser Protein Source
Almonds and Almond butter	Peanuts and peanut butter
Quinoa	Green beans & any large, starchy bean: kidney, great northern, lima
Tempeh	Tofu and "mock meats"
Organic, plain, European (Greek) yogurt	Regular yogurt
Organic DHA-enhanced eggs	Egg substitute and/or regular eggs
Tuna fish	Fish sticks and popcorn shrimp
Wild salmon	Farmed salmon
Organic chicken	Regular frozen chicken
Grass-fed beef	Grain-fed beef

Humans can produce half of the twenty amino acids, but the others must be supplied by the diet. Failure to obtain enough of even one of the essential amino acids results in erosion of the body's proteins. Exactly which amino acids are essential, and how many, can be disputed, since some amino acids are made from others. Therefore, if a particular amino acid is present in the body, another one may be synthesized, but if the first is missing, then both are deficient.

Both whole food and supplemental proteins are necessary to achieve a complete nutritional balance as well as the desired level of protein intake. Protein is the only one of the three basic macronutrients that can be used as it is needed. While protein cannot become an *essential* fatty acid, protein can also be used either as a common fatty acid or as a carbohydrate.

> *Protein's denaturation can be reversible or irreversible, depending upon its environment.*

Protein Denaturation

Cooking changes the molecular structure and characteristics of protein; enzymes are basically proteins, too. Here is what happens: the most complicated—power-packed—form of protein is called quaternary form—taking on the appearance of highly connected interwoven spirals and twists. The simplest form is the primary form, much like a string of pearls in a necklace with the pearls being the amino acids (see the table, Proteins and their Structure, page 223). There are two other forms in between but we will not discuss them here. The point is that when proteins and enzymes are heated they denature, or their connections loosen up from the highly bound quaternary form to the loosely held primary form, and that is not nutritionally good. Some of these changes may be reversible but others are not, so these compromised amino acids become unusable.

Protein denaturation can be caused by heating or freezing, pH change, changes in the concentration of other substances (like salts, acids and/or alkaline substances, etc.) dissolved in any surrounding fluids, and by other processes like ultrasonic stress and aging. This is one of the main reasons why it is necessary for humans (and other animals) to maintain a stable temperature and pH.

Protein in Your Diet

> *Consuming enough protein each day is the dietary key to ensuring the weight you lose is fat and NOT muscle.*

People of all ages and activity levels need a complete protein source. Our bodies can make about half of the needed amino acids, so they must be present in our diets in a specific ratio to each other. So if a person does not get enough of one of them to match with the rest, the rest can only be used at a level to balance with that low one; this results in a deficiency.

> *When you are on the go, protein powders, meal replacements, protein bars, and protein snacks are convenient and they taste good.*

Amino acids are only used to the extent of the least one that is available, and if that one is heat labile—sensitive to heat degradation—then that essential component for repair is unavailable, not only compromising the protein structure, but also anywhere that same protein might be needed and used in the entire body.

Most of these amino acids are fairly easy to consume in a reasonably well-balanced diet. However, there are a few amino acids that are a little harder to obtain than the rest, thus it is important to make sure you are eating enough of them. If any individual or combinations of these *limiting amino acids* are deficient in a person's diet, this will limit the usefulness of all the others, even if those others are present in otherwise large enough quantities. The limiting amino acids include the sulfur-containing amino acids (methionine and cysteine), tryptophan, and lysine. Interestingly, one of the most heat labile amino acids is lysine, the other being threonine.

Proper Protein Intake

My suggestion is for patients to consume one gram of protein powder for every kilogram (2.2 pounds) of body weight. Generally, the average person should consume between 0.8g to 1.7 g of protein per kilogram of body weight, depending on their lean body weight, their fitness goals, and their lifestyle. The more active a person is, the more protein that person requires. So an adult male who weighs 195 pounds should divide his body weight by 2.2 to find out how many grams of protein he should eat. Well, that is too much math for most people, so to find the ballpark answer I tell my patients to divide their body weight by 2. Answer: 93 kilograms, the same as the number of protein grams they should eat each day.

Many people believe that they must eat meat to get their protein, but this is not true! Besides, cooking protein is not good for the protein's quality. Consume the equivalent in a plant-based protein source and eat the other proteins if you like, even perhaps a combination of the two for insurance.

Protein Supplementation

Did you know that the desire for something sweet, like sugar, is a sign of a protein deficiency? When I find that my patients have a sweet tooth, one of the first nutrients I check is protein because eating more protein will cure a sugar craving.

While protein powders and meal replacements make good economic sense, they are meant to supplement the diet. It is still important to eat whole foods because whole foods provide the essential components for tissue repair that are not found in man-made nutrients.

When you think of protein, consider drinking a protein supplement that at least supplies your essential amino acids; optimally it will meet all your protein needs. A protein drink is a quicker and much more convenient version of protein-rich foods.

The highest PDCAAS is found in some of the "mainstream" protein sources: casein, whey, egg, and soy protein. Rice, one of the least offensive grains, has a PDCAAS of 0.47, followed by hemp at 0.46.

When I ask patients about where they obtain their protein, they regularly answer me by saying that they eat some sort of cooked flesh—red meat, poultry, or fish—dairy or eggs. When I follow up by asking them how much protein they consume in a day, I hear crickets. In most cases, people are unaware that proteins are broken down by heat that generally exceeds body temperature, nor do they know how much protein they need to consume daily to maintain their health.

As a result of their ignorance, if the essential amino acids—most often those amino acids that are most heat labile—are unavailable in a person's diet, then some other amino acid will have to take the place of the one that is missing in the long amino acid chains that make up proteins. These are the same proteins that make up neurochemicals, neurotransmitters, hormones and the like, and therefore, when an amino acid chain changes, so does that protein's function. This change is akin to the brain speaking in a bizarre dialect of neurologese. Who can understand it?

Whey is the most popular protein supplement because it is the fastest digesting; casein is the slowest. Casein is an ideal choice when you deliberately want protein to digest slowly, like during the day as part of any normal meal. Further, when whey protein is combined with a meal containing carbs, fat and/or other nutrients, the digestion of whey slows down to the point where it's likely just as suitable as casein for those meals. Finally, since you usually spend seven to eight hours nightly in a fasted state, it makes a lot of sense to consume a casein source of protein before you go to bed. It helps your body recover and repair from the day's activities.

Summary

A healthy nervous system depends on one area knowing exactly what another area is doing. A functional brain must have an internal communication so it can behave as a well-timed unit with each part synchronizing with each of the other parts, which includes the spinal cord and peripheral nerves—that's neurologese.

To be effective in today's world of alternative health, a doctor must be fluent in neurologese. It is a very specific language—a functional blend of structure and behavior—based on performance and timing that ultimately displays the coincidence of neurological events, even though they may seem unrelated to one another. When the doctor understands neurologese, he or she can converse with the nervous system, make a few corrections and bring about changes that appear almost miraculous.

If your brain has lost its words, get them back! Find a doctor who knows how to help your brain reestablish the nervous system's timing; one who can return the neurological signals to their proper spinal cord and brain targets, to bring about the right NTs that stimulate the brain to its pre-designed expression.

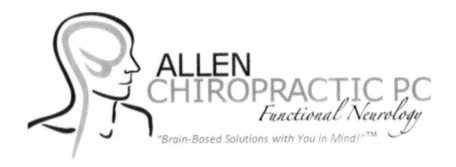

ALLEN
CHIROPRACTIC PC
Functional Neurology

"Brain-Based Solutions with You in Mind!"™

SECTION IV

"STOP THE STATIC!"

CHAPTER EIGHT

IF YOUR BRAIN COULD SPEAK, IT MIGHT SAY...

"Stop the Static!"

Now that we have learned the importance of proper nutrition for better brain health, let's turn our focus to the nerves, spinal cord, and the nerve signals that create better brain function.

What happens in the nerves, spinal cord, and brain when their neurological signals get "staticky"? Nerves detest interference because it confuses the overall scheme of things. "Static" denotes nerve signals that are mistimed relative to the other signals that surround them.

Certain nerves (proprioceptors) provide a sensory input from muscles, tendons, and joints giving the central nervous system an unconscious perception of the body's position in space (proprioception—proh·pree·o·sep·shuhn). They envelop a joint and are motion sensitive. When these

Definition: Staticky
• *Relating to or producing random noise accompanying transmitted or recorded sound;*
• *Relating to or producing electrostatic charges;*
• *Affected by random noise due to electrical interference: staticky radio reception.*

259

nerves perceive even the slightest movement, they ignite signals to the cord, then on to the brain reaching it almost instantly. Proprioceptors send their signals to the brain at 120 meters per second. That is greater than the length of one and one-third football fields in one second. *That's fast!* The brain processes all this input just as fast and sends its motor response back down to the cord and out to the muscles to complete the cycle so the joints and muscles move as one synchronous and functional unit.

> *When one muscle group does work, coordinated groups must oppose that work for the sum of the action to equal zero.*

By design, muscles that move a joint should pull with balance and counterbalance. The brain depends upon the interaction of muscle activity for its stimulation. When one muscle works, another one that offsets it has to release its pull so the first one can complete its cycle. This functional interplay goes on every split second of every day, and when it fails, so does joint stability. This balanced movement is the key to optimal human performance. But not just any movement will do; it has to be *reciprocal* movement.

Reciprocal movement sends clear nerve signals to the cord and brain. Nerve static occurs whenever there is uncoordinated, disconnected, or mismatched movement. Nerve static baffles the cord and brain; it makes them do things they should not do and not do things they should do. This displays as muscles that turn off when they should be on, and are on when they should be off.

Static compromises joint integrity and static leads to structural instability. Movement patterns emerge that appear to be contrary to their original intent. One might say that these movement patterns were "other-than-human" because the human system is suboptimal when these pat-

> *When you bend your arm, your biceps contract and your triceps reciprocate by stretching. One muscle contracts while the other stretches.*
>
> *The actions of the muscles are opposite but the amount is equal.*

terns arise. Further, since these dysfunctional movements are different than their original intention, it makes these signals pathological, eventually leading to more serious problems.

If your brain could speak, it would probably say, "I'm getting mixed signals!"

In previous chapters, we have learned that the brain gives top priority to input from muscles and joints. So while nutrition is important to brain function—it keeps the brain healthy, willing, and able to send and receive sig-

> *A muscle that stabilizes a joint in preparation for movement is called a "shunt" muscle; it holds a joint steady so that movement can take place. The mover is called a "spurt" muscle. Its action causes motion.*

nals—let's not forget the importance of the signal itself. Since the brain gives top priority to the signals received from the muscles and joints, let's make sure our bodies are not sending weak, degraded, "staticky" messages.

> *When a muscle "turns on" it is said to be functionally facilitated. When it "turns off" it is said to be functionally inhibited. Facilitation and inhibition are neurological words that describe the state of the nerve signal relative to their control centers.*

Muscles work according to a preprogrammed set of neurologic motor sequences. For example, in order for a joint like the elbow to flex and extend smoothly, several muscles have to coordinate that movement. Let's just consider two of these muscles that op-

pose each other. When muscle number one contracts—as in flexion, or curling at the elbow—muscle number two is preprogrammed to relax proportional to the increased work of muscle number one, which is doing its job of curling the elbow. Muscle number two cannot work against muscle number one if the elbow is going to flex properly; muscle number two counterbalances elbow flexion. Conversely, when the elbow extends, muscle number one must now relax so that muscle number two can do its work to straighten the elbow back out again. This reciprocal exchange idea is true for any joint movement.

When one muscle contracts, the one that opposes the movement cannot also contract or the joint stiffens, and the end result is potential damage. If both muscles tried to work at the same time, the joint would bind up and lead to terrible elbow problems over time, like joint stiffness, aches and pains, general discomfort; the joint would probably become arthritic. This is true for movement in any part of the body—front to back, side to side, and top to bottom.

Muscles are designed to contract, and each one must pull its weight to the best of its ability. Each muscle has its own job to do; some stabilize while others cause movement. One muscle cannot possibly do the work of two. Even the same muscle on opposite sides of the body has a different function. Although they look the same from one side to the other, they pull differently—they are mirror images of each other.

For Every Action...

The proper management of joint motion is called "reciprocity." Reciprocity requires coordination and strategy that can only come from a static-free nervous system. Theoretically, the sum of all the joint forces that come into play when its muscles do work should equal zero. When one muscle works another must relax; the sum is balance.

The Tonic Neck Reflex
Turning the head to one side causes the facilitation of extensor muscles toward that same side and the facilitation of flexor muscles on the opposite side.

There are shunt muscles and there are spurt muscles. Shunt muscles stabilize the joint so that the spurt muscles can move it. Again, back to the elbow example: In order for the elbow to flex, certain shunt muscles must stabilize the arm so that the spurt muscles can move the bones of the forearm. For the elbow to avoid damage, shunt muscles hold the joint while the reciprocal spurt mechanisms of flexion versus extension, for example, work together to cancel each other out.

When muscles work other than reciprocally—when their movements clash rather than coordinate—and their sum is anything other than zero, their display is other-than-human. Looking back at our elbow example, when muscle number one has a bit more tone than muscle number two, which opposes the stronger muscle, the elbow is biased to curl. Let's take our example a step further. Every time muscle number two tries to overcome muscle number one to straighten the elbow, the stronger muscle—number one—tends to prevail, increasing the tendency for elbow strain and injury. Contentious motion is an indication that the brain's input and output systems are full of static, or confused.

"Let's consider shoulder joint motion. Raise your arm out to your side and up to the level of your shoulder. Before your arm can move at the shoulder joint, other muscles must first stabilize the shoulder blade and the rest of the shoulder

In general, the brain's input comes from the opposite side of the body. The right side of the brain receives input from the left side of the body and the left side of the brain receives input from the right side of the body.

girdle. When the shoulder blade is still, for example, the arm can move on top of the stable shoulder blade. In this case we say that there is spurt motion of the arm upon a properly shunted shoulder blade. Now, when you continue your arm's motion through that same range of motion and up overhead, the previously shunted shoulder blade must now take on a spurt motion and the stability of the shoulder girdle moves more centrally to the spine. This way the whole shoulder girdle can move in its preprogrammed manner.

However, if any of the shoulder blade stabilizers become sloppy— taking on erroneous movement where the muscles turn off when they should be on, and on when they should be off, or when they shunt when they should spurt or vice versa—the arm movement at the shoulder becomes sloppy too, and these muscle problems ultimately lead to shoulder joint pain and joint breakdown; i.e., a frozen shoulder, for example. Further, since all sensory signals ultimately reach the brain, the brain suffers, too. This is an excellent example of neurological static; *deafferentation*."

Deafferentation has some of its most powerful effects when the muscles of the spine lose their shunt stability. All the muscles within the spinal column and that support spinal movement are antigravity muscles. Antigravity muscles are designed to stand us upright and endure the effects of gravity 24 hours a day, 7 days a week. Each of these spinal muscles should be full of ATP, which enables continual work. When the centerline spine—the axial skeleton—breaks down and is no longer able to shunt and/or spurt according to their original neurological plan, there is nowhere else to find stability and the structure suffers as a whole.

Static in the Nerve Channels

> *If the archer's muscles turned on contrary to their original design, which is quite commonly found in clinical practice, then the muscles would be sending conflicting signals to the brain indicating that the head turned the other way.*

Now, since it is the muscles that generate the brain's highest priority signals, any erroneous muscle function will eventually lead to functional brain problems. These signaling errors lead to *static* in the nervous system. This static leads to confusion, making it hard for the brain to "hear" what is really happening and confounding its response to it.

Here is another example: Turing the head to one side normally causes the muscles of extension to turn on toward the side of head rotation and turn off on the other side. (Imagine an archer's posture.) This is normal human programming called the *tonic neck reflex* (TNR). If, however, the muscles work backwards—that is, if the flexors turn on toward the side of head rotation, and/or the extensors turn off on that same side—then static reaches the brain and its control centers, making them either do things they should not be doing or not do things they should be doing. Aberrant muscle input creates an aberrant motor response. There are many other physiological examples where nerve function sets up signaling errors in the brain and spinal cord.

A Bitter Pill

Motor planning problems, ADD, ADHD, depression, etc., are generally treated with medications, but medicines just cover up the mismatched signals by sedating one area or stimulating another in ways unlike their original programming. Drugs do nothing to resolve the

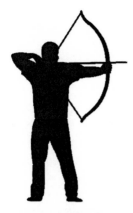

**An Archer Depicts
the Tonic Neck Reflex
Posture**

problem; the brain just "tunes out" the static. Tuning out the static is not the same as eliminating its source.

Most parents are against medicating their learning-disabled children, but they are often times not given other satisfactory options by their medical doctors. The truth is that effective alternatives do exist that are non-invasive and grounded in medical research, which is more solid than the so-called "benefits" of medication. Unfortunately, during the course of a child's treatment, one medication is often switched to a second or third as their benefits wear off over time.

Drugs and medications overwrite their own programs upon a dysfunctional brain, making its functions drift further and further from its original programming. There may be small changes, but the overall brain performance consistently suffers. While medications can affect specific nerve centers, they cannot focus on one side of the brain or any of its many vital centers without simultaneously affecting all the others. Medications bathe the entire brain with effects that eventually create behaviors contrary to its programming. Further, many of the most common medications are not tested for use by children, and their long term effects have never been studied. Some are known to create problems in nerve cell function, and others may lead to brain cancers. They change the way neurochemicals work, either making them hang around longer or eliminating them faster. They change the timing in the nerve's on/off switches, but at what price? Most of the time the hidden costs are not known until much later and the bill comes due with more complicated behaviors, sickness and disease.

Coordination and Learning

Most people are aware that the right and left sides of the brain are different both anatomically and functionally. Each side is naturally influenced by how well muscles and joints do their jobs. Regarding the brain's incoming signals, each half of the brain generally receives input from the muscles and joints on the opposite side of the body.

The muscle and joint signals from one side of the body generally influence the function of the cortex on the opposite side. Concerning the outgoing signals from the brain, each side of the brain similarly controls the muscle

> *Every muscle has its optimal pull when its origin and insertion are at their most favorable distance apart. If the origin and insertion become too far apart or too close together, the muscle fatigues.*

and joint motion on the opposite side of the body. In general, the communication signals—both incoming and outgoing—switch between the side of the brain and the side of the body. (There are fundamental exceptions to this rule, but their explanation might only serve to complicate the picture, so simplicity is important here.)

If muscles fatigue either because they have worked too hard or the joints they influence have become stuck, then the number of incoming signals to the brain withers. This is another example of what we call *deafferentation*. When the brain becomes deafferentated, communication errors begin, one side of the brain works harder than the other, and learning suffers.

Further, it is quite common for people to have more problems on one side of their body than the other. That sets up a deafferentation bias, resulting in mismatched signals to and from the brain. This disparity is known as hemisphericity, and it is fundamental to learning problems. Have you ever noticed that people with learning problems also seem to have movement troubles? Coordination and learning go hand in hand.

> *Certain anti-depressants have been known to cause children to become irritable, restless, impulsive, agitated, aggressive, and unclear in their thinking.*

While muscle signals generally reach the brain on the opposite side, muscle signals uniquely also go to the same side cerebellum. Both muscle and joint signals go to the thalamus and brain on the side opposite to their origin, but *the cerebellum only receives input from muscles on the same side as their origin*; the cerebellum receives no input from the joints themselves. When the cerebellum and thalamus collect all the incoming information—including that from the special senses, such as touch, vision, hearing, and taste (remember, smell is different)—it gets sent to the rest of the brain, and that sets the stage for the brain's synchronization.

However, if one side of the brain is working better than the other, does it make sense to treat both sides with drugs or just the side causing the problems? Would you cast both arms if only one was broken? Certainly not. Then why give someone a drug that has no selective ability to affect one side of the brain over the other? Medicines affect both sides of the brain; they have no way of selecting only one focal area with a problem and leaving the functional areas unaffected. Therefore, the best way to influence brain performance is to diagnose the one area of the brain needing help and then treat that area with non-invasive measures. Medications can not do that.

The brain's timing patterns are intimately sensitive to muscle and joint movements. When the muscles and joints move freely, clearer nerve signals are sent to the brain's timing centers. That generates the neurochemicals specific to that area, and they regulate their own production without the need for drugs or medications. The brain is the ultimate regulator of physiological processes.

The appropriate movement patterns unlock the ability to learn because reciprocal movements send the right signals to each side of the brain, and the brain can respond more appropriately. And since the most important signals to the brain come from the centerline skeleton—those centerline structures that are higher up are more important than those that are lower down—proper signal motion is essential to static-free brain function. This idea of functional reciprocity is one of the keys to understanding just what each person's nervous system needs in order for that person to perform at their highest level.

Cortical Character Traits

Left Brain	Right Brain
Male traits	Female traits
Logical	Random
Sequential	Feelings
Rational	Intuitive
Analytical	Holistic
Feeling	Synthesizing
Objective	Subjective
Detail oriented	"Big picture" oriented
Facts rule	Imagination rules
Words & Language	Symbols & Images
Present & Past	Present & Future
Math & Science	Philosophy & Religion
Can comprehend	Can "Get it"
Knowing	Believing
Acknowledges	Appreciates
Order/Pattern Perception	Spatial perception
Knows object's name	Knows object's function
Reality-based	Fantasy-based
Forms strategies	Presents possibilities
Practical	Impetuous
Predictable	Takes risks

Drugs, such as stimulants, anti-depressants, painkillers, muscle re-laxers, etc., may temporarily take away anxiety, discomfort or pain, but do not allow yourself to be fooled. Drugs and medications are another source of static. They immerse the entire body in their effects and side effects. There are alternatives. In many cases, nerve static can be located with just a simple neurological examination to analyze personal habits—dietary choices, exercise routine, sleep patterns, stress, etc.—and treated with functional therapies. Functional neurology coupled with applied kinesiology does just that.

Reducing Your Brain's Static Cling

Your brain is built for change. Every nerve signal that reaches the spinal cord and brain ultimately influences how the brain works. My job is to help influence it for the better. Further, and almost without exception, every brain input ultimately finds its expression in the contraction of a muscle. So it makes sense that doing exercise and other activities of daily living—linked to your individual needs—often enough will generate more nerve signals along a specific path, and that changes the way your brain works.

> *The hemispheric model theorizes that one side of the brain is not firing properly, generally having a different level of function. This is usually due to a reduced level of stimulation caused by a joint position error (e.g., vertebral subluxation) or some other neurological problem. Essentially, if one neurological system is not firing properly, then all those neurological systems subsequent to it will also not fire properly.*

As a nerve impulse travels the length of a nerve, it eventually reaches a synapse—like a relay station; the gap or space between one nerve and the next—causing the release of neurochemicals into the gap. Those neurochemicals respond best when they are stimulated according to the right frequency and timing, and they, in turn, are better able to stimulate the next nerve. The signal continues to that nerve's eventual end where the cycle repeats. Generally, the more often a nerve is stimulated, the greater will be the release of its neurochemicals at the nerve's end—the terminal end, or *bouton terminal*. This builds plasticity into the system. Further, a single nerve may have its effect on another single nerve, but more probably one nerve can affect as many as thousands of other nerves as their signals spread throughout the entire nervous system.

> *According to most studies, the human brain stops growing in its early 20s, after which it starts to contract. But new studies show as we age it is never too late to begin a brain workout and that it can make a difference.*

Nature encourages neurochemicals to linger in the synapse because the synapse does not receive much blood at all that could wash the neurochemicals away. The paucity of blood encourages the persistence of neurochemicals, which allows more nerve signals to cross over to the next nerve. More neurochemicals means more nerve signals, which means greater "plasticity."

Change Your Brain, Change Your Health

Plasticity is a non-specific neurological concept that emphasizes the brain is not static and will, in fact, respond to new learning. It expresses the ability of the brain and nervous system to change structurally and functionally as a result of input from the environment. Generally, plasticity denotes the ability for neurological transformation. When a nerve fires a signal through the spinal cord, it readies another nerve to fire its signals, too. By design, these signals reach the front part of the spinal cord (see, Schematic of the Spinal Cord and Nerves, located on page 270) and result in an expected series of muscle responses that both support and move the involved joint. Certain muscles should turn on and others should turn off in a predictable and orchestrated synchrony according to a preset plan. These same signals also fire upward to the brain, making several connections along the way, and then return again to the spinal cord to help modify the cord's coordinated response. But, because of the interplay of neurological dynamics, these nerve signals can become confused, causing disorder that can lead to erroneous muscle displays. This is where the nervous system and its reciprocity become tongue-tied.

> *Medications are unable to pinpoint a dysfunctional brain center. Rather, drug side effects can happen at sites distant from their intent because they work systemically.*

These persistent, inappropriate responses can become the "new norm" that cause the brain to integrate these mismatched signals into the particular neurological pathways,

> *Researchers find that physical exercise may slow the effects of aging and help people maintain cognitive abilities well into older age.*

which express movement patterns that are other than those that would be considered normal. That too is plasticity, but it is dysplasticity. Dysplasticity is less efficient and pathological because it is not neuro-typical. Negative plasticity cannot be supported by normal physiological processes, so while

> *Brain fitness is like physical fitness. Some is better than none, and more is better than some, according to researchers.*

its signals can express themselves, they cannot be sustained and at the same time be healthy. Because it is quite likely that somewhere along the path these nerve signals negatively affect muscle and joint function, it is highly probable that the involved muscles work for a very short period and then fatigue—and when these muscles fatigue

> *Sustaining physical fitness, good nutrition, a vibrant social life, plus brain fitness will enable successful aging.*

they do so in spasm, because it takes calcium for a muscle to contract and ATP energy for a muscle to relax—leading to a greater likelihood of joint breakdown with an increased potential for injury.

To maximize your brain's functional abilities, doesn't it make more sense to redirect the process and cause the incoming signals to go where they are designed to go and keep dysplasticity from interrupting that process? It sounds easy enough, but how is it done?

Most people turn to nutritional supplements to change the way their body works. But while nutrition plays a vital role in brain health—just as it does in hormone production, pain management, and energy formation—nutrients are not the best way to stimulate the brain. Remember, the brain's primary stimulation comes from the input related to muscles and joints. Therefore, any stimulus other than the primary stimulus has a secondary

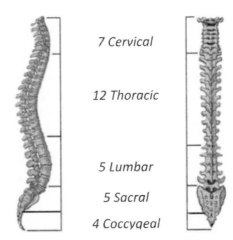

7 Cervical

12 Thoracic

5 Lumbar

5 Sacral

4 Coccygeal

The Spine, its Various Vertebrae, and its Landmarks

effect on the brain's performance. The very best way to stimulate the brain is to give it the input it craves—specific exercises, reciprocal motion, physical rehabilitation, coupled adjustments, etc.—and its needs are expressed in "neurologese."

The Cord is a Happening Place!

The spinal cord is very orderly. It must be organized because nerve signals enter and leave the cord at lightning speeds. Simply put, the spinal cord is a very busy place.

The Cord's Design

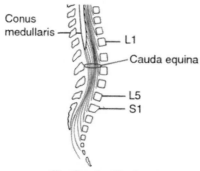

The Caudae Equina

The spinal column and spinal cord are different. The adult spinal column (see "The Spine, its Various Vertebrae, and its Landmarks," pictured on page 271) consists of the vertebrae that make up the spine—twenty-six in all, consisting of the following: 7 cervical, 12 thoracic (dorsal), 5 lumbar, 1 sacral (5 sacral segments that naturally fuse together as one), and 1 coccygeal (4 coccygeal segments that naturally fuse together as one) vertebrae. The spinal cord is part of the central nervous system—together with the brain—that functions primarily in the transmission of neural signals up and down the cord, between the brain and the rest of the body. Its neural circuitry can independently control several different reflexes and manage the nerve pathways that program movement patterns.

The spinal cord is divided into thirty-one different segments, each designed for order and efficiency, connecting the peripheral nervous system to the brain. The spinal cord is housed within a bony canal made up of the adjoining vertebrae, and runs from the base of the skull to the junction between the twelfth thoracic and first lumbar vertebra (i.e., T12 and L1). From there, the nerves that come off the spinal cord are called the caudae equina, because they look like a horse's tail.

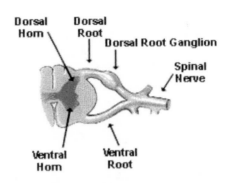

Schematic of the Spinal Cord and Nerves

For each nerve signal that enters the *dorsal horn* of each spinal cord segment (the back part of the cord; see the diagram to the right), twelve different but intimately involved synapses occur. That is, once an individual nerve signal reaches the incoming part of the spinal cord, it stimulates twelve different individual reactions each having its own effect. Each segment of the spinal cord contributes its own preprogrammed influence for the overall order and efficiency of the spinal cord. Its hierarchical effect is organized from upper to lower—from cervical to coccygeal segments.

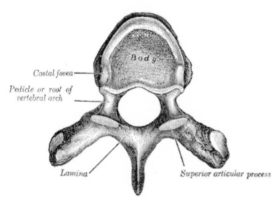

A Typical Vertebra Showing the Spinal Canal

This hierarchical design makes the cord a happening place; and nobody can count how many nerve signals enter the cord at any one time—it is immeasurable. Each segment contributes to its own survival, by influencing the management of glucose and oxygen, inhibiting nociception, and sending connecting signals up and down the cord between the involved segment and the brain. These first four influences make up 33% of the twelve responses. The other 67% of the reactions to an individual nerve signal involve the muscles.

Within each cord segment, the remaining eight segmental influences coordinate prearranged muscle function related to that segment, and intermix with the others in two to three segment increments, entwining the segments for maximum efficiency. Those eight influences are divided into four sets of two, each. Two sets of two relate to the upper extremities, and the other two sets of two relate to the lower extremities in order to manage the preprogrammed human movement patterns. Each cord segment contains these centers for preprogrammed reciprocal movement patterns.

> *If the human nervous system is designed to cause muscles to perform in a predetermined manner, then any muscle display other than that design must be contrary to the human schematic; it is "other-than-human."*

And if all this neurological order is true for the cord it must also be true for the brain. But while the nervous system's setup is one thing, sadly such is not always true when it comes to its function. The pathways may be symmetrical, but the signals that go through them can become mismatched. Asymmetrical or unbalanced spinal cord and/or brain signals functionally confound their orderly design; the tracts themselves do not change, but the signals they convey do.

The Effects of Unbalanced Cord Signals

The *ventral horn* (the front part of the cord; see diagram, page 273) is the last spinal center that can influence the motor signals as they leave the cord. It is called the final common pathway, because it is where all the motor signals come together; from the brain above, the segments around, and the cord below. The name fits because all nerve signals must pass through this last corridor before they can do their jobs. For our purposes, we will discuss the ventral horn's influence on muscles.

> *Two of the brain's major timing centers are the cerebellum and thalamus. These two areas must be in sync with each other in order for the brain to perform optimally.*

In a perfect world, if all the input to the final common pathway is in sync, then the muscles will be balanced. However—because nothing in this world is ever perfect—everyone has some aspect of structural imbalance. It is a neurological expectation that more signals reach the brain from one side of the body than the other. This asymmetry sets up mismatched brain signals, but it is the nervous system's forté to manage these imbalances and make sense of them. Nevertheless, the accumulation of neurological error gradually compromises even these intricate control systems, allowing mismanaged control signals to reach the final common pathway, leading to timing errors—another form of static. All these brain signals, balanced or not, ultimately have an effect on the muscles.

Static in the cord is like a computer that cannot process data fast enough and becomes bogged down. When the ventral horn signals cannot update themselves fast enough, the muscles tend to pull when they should relax, or relax when they should pull—and that unbalances the structure.

Imagine what happens in the cord when chaotic signals fly around without restraint. The functional human nervous system is not meant to work in a disorganized manner, and any muscles that contract or relax in a style contrary to their original programming display an "other-than-human" character.

Gravity and the Human Nervous System

Unfortunately, varying degrees of confused nerve signals occur in almost every patient I see. When people ask me how this happens, my answer is "gravity." Gravity is everywhere. At every moment, gravity is the force that the human system fights to overcome. It is the silent complication that makes the human system express its unique character.

The human nervous system thrives on a changing environment, one that is balanced and has plenty of input from moving joints and working muscles and a minimal amount of static interference. However, any muscle dysfunction that generates staticky nerve signals often leads to central nervous system dysfunction, circuitry breakdown, and general sickness. When nerve static persists, it eventually leads to muscle and joint problems, lower energy, accelerated aging,

Understanding "Neurologese"

"Neurologese" is the primary language of the brain. Although it might seem complicated, it is relatively easy to understand because the brain expresses what it needs and its needs are obvious, if you know what to look for and how to interpret it. One of my teachers, the late George Goodheart, DC, taught me that the human nervous system is intricately simple and simply intricate. He was right.

Reflexes

When you sit on the doctor's table and he or she strikes your knee with a reflex hammer, your thigh jerks, and your foot kicks. That is the patellar reflex and this display is normal. The same thing should happen on the other knee, too. Tendon stimulation reflexively leads to muscle contraction. That same response can happen to any tendon and muscle. These reflexes are physiological—they are built into, and are an intimate part of the human design. (Various tendon reflexes are very clinically useful.)

There are other physiological reflexes of varying complexity, and their names usually indicate what they do. One of them is the tonic neck reflex (TNR). It has to do with neck muscle tone and function.

Turning the head to the right, for example, excites the same side muscles of extension (those that take the extremities away from the body), while simultaneously inhibiting the right muscles of flexion (those that bring the extremities closer to the body). Reflexes must have this reciprocal function so joints can move properly. Meanwhile, the muscles on the side opposite the head rotation—those on the left side—respond in the opposite way; the muscles work reciprocally. That is, when the head turns to the right, the left-sided extensor muscles should be inhibited (or turned off) while the left-sided flexors should be facilitated (or turned on). This is what we would expect to see according to the normal human design, but it does not always happen like that.

The books say these TNRs go away after a certain age. Actually, they become integrated with other reflexes to create the fabric of our human movement patterns. When these reflexes are in sync the static is gone, but when they get confused the static is deafening to the cord and brain, and normal nerve responses get overrun.

and a higher probability of pain. Uncorrected disorder begets disorder, and persistent disorder quickly and silently becomes trapped in a vicious cycle leading to pathologies like arthritis, fibromyalgia, and many other chronic debilitating diseases.

Timing Errors Can Cause Trauma

All humans have the same nerve pathways. Everyone's nervous system is the same anatomically, but each of us uses our nervous system differently, and that is good because these individuations are what makes each of us unique.

Some people use their right hand and others use their left hand more. The neurological pathways to and from either hand are symmetrical, yet people use them differently. Further, the more we use one hand relative to the other the more we sculpt our nervous system relative to how we use it. We increase the plasticity along the pathways of highest use while we simultaneously sculpt away the unused pathways. We shape our nervous systems to make them even more unique through both use and disuse. Plasticity, both good and bad, sculpts our personality, structure, and identity. The saying, "Use it or lose it" applies nicely when it comes to the plastic human nervous system.

The more signals that cross a nerve pathway, the greater is the probability that the signals will develop plasticity—they will persist. Nerve signals that are more stimulated become more grooved. This can be good if the functionally proper signals are being reinforced along the proper pathways; but bad if the wrong signals are being reinforced. Functional or not, the more signals that travel along any given nerve pathway the more normal these avenues become for these signals. This is neurological learning.

Learning and Experience are All about Timing

The brain is the ultimate processing center. Different areas of the brain have their own specific and unique rhythm in order to conserve energy. At various times, certain centers are normally "on,"

> *All sensory input ultimately has its display in the contraction of a muscle.*

and others are normally "off." When a system is "on," it is receptive, and when it is "off," it rests. Before two centers can share information, the nervous system that connects them must be "on" and receptive. The problem is that not all centers are "on" at the same time. Brain centers can only work when they are switched "on."

Even a simple arm movement follows this same rule. Although your brain instinctively knows how to stabilize a joint in order to make a particular movement, the motor system must wait for its controllers to be "on" before any movement can happen. The same idea applies to learning.

> *Learning is like an ant colony. Each ant has its own job but together they help the colony survive and grow. Similarly, our experiences help us learn.*

The Deep Tendon Reflex (DTR)

The deep tendon reflex is a clinical tool to evaluate spinal cord function. It is a stretch reflex that displays the consistency of a reflex arc between the spinal cord and brain areas that innervate the muscle.

The sensory (incoming) part of the reflex begins with the instantaneous stretch of the muscle's tendon. The impulse enters the dorsal horn where the information takes four routes. It enters the dorsal horn and: 1) it synapses directly on a motor neuron, which causes immediate contraction of the muscle innervated by that receptor, the primary mover; 2) it synapses on an inhibitory neuron that then synapses on a motor neuron that goes to a muscle opposed to the primary mover causing an associated relaxation of the second muscle as the primary muscle contracts. The impulse also mixes with other tracts that arise to the: 3) cerebellum, and 4) cortex.

The signals that reach the cerebellum and cortex turn around and descend again to exert a controlling influence over the activities in the ventral horn of the cord.

We learn and gain experience by taking in information, but the data has no meaning unless it can be connected and used by the brain. It is not enough to have stockpiled vast stores of data around the brain in various places. Every single moment is priceless to our human experience but what good is it if it is unlinked with another moment? Linking data is the key to learning and experience. These data caches must be able to talk to one another. Interpretation of our experiences is done both consciously and unconsciously. Interpretation is what blends every conscious and unconscious experience into a unified whole so that we can learn more about our environment.

Two seemingly separate bits of datum can be connected if the centers that deal with the data are switched "on" at the same time. When these streams of input are coupled, they can be related to memory.

Gravity Happens!

My eldest brother, Barney, came to see me for treatment one day with a sharp knee pain. I asked him what happened, and he said he was walking down the street, turned a corner and was, "surprised by a gravity storm." He fell down! Gravity got the best of him and down he went.

I thought that was a great word picture. "Gravity happens," and it happens to each of us daily. The truth is, we may not fall down, but our bodies know that gravity has its way with us.

Gravity is one of life's constants. If you think about the human nervous system you will realize that it cannot persist without gravity; we subconsciously wrestle against it every day. Gravity is that stimulus that makes us express one of our basic human traits—upright posture. Even space travelers need gravity to stay healthy.

Gravity is not just a matter of up and down. Rather, gravity is that attraction that constantly tugs against our frame; it also makes us stand on two feet. Our body's ability to resist gravity is directly related to our degree of neurological wellness. Appropriate functional reflexes indicate a healthy spinal cord and brain, but reflex dysfunction is an indicator of static in the spinal cord and brain. All of us, including me, need a fully healthy nervous system.

Humans are the only species to resist gravity on two feet. The ability to stand upright is a function of the cerebellum. Consider the infant on his or her belly, who lifts their head to see the world. From that point on, gravity is the antagonist of the human nervous system. Every movement thereafter is calculated relative to gravity.

We all have our own center of gravity (COG). It is like a circle that surrounds us wherever we go. The circles of some people are larger than those of others because people's balance varies. The healthier we are, the more we tend to stay within our circle. If we venture outside that circle, we tend to stumble, and sometimes we fall. Those who only stumble often catch themselves without falling down because their reflexes keep them upright against the attraction of gravity. Did you know that the leading cause of accidental death is the incidental fall? Absolutely true!

Reflexes work outside our reasoning—like an instinct. If we had to stop and think about not falling after we stumble, we would fall instantly because gravity is faster than our thoughts, therefore, we are designed to respond reflexively. Reflexes are preprogrammed for specific responses to gravity.

However, if these two bits of information arrive at their destination at the same time, but the center is in its "off" mode, the center is unable to process the data and the signals can go no further. A stream of dead end data means virtually nothing. It is as if the data died for lack of a linkage.

The flexor withdrawal reflex (also called a nociceptive or flexor withdrawal response) is a spinal reflex intended to protect the body from damaging stimuli, like touching something hot. The reflex facilitates specific flexor muscles and inhibits specific extensor muscles, characterized by abrupt withdrawal of a body part in response to painful stimulation.

Even a puff of air across the eyeball causes a protective blink response. And a grumble in the stomach may be because of a gas bubble that passes a specific receptor. Every time a receptor is stimulated there is some kind of muscular response, and that response has a meaning if the observer understands it. The point is that every signal that reaches and is processed by the brain ultimately expresses itself in the contraction of some kind of muscle.

The whole experience of data input and processing, and the response to that processing—the motor response—can be measured using applied kinesiology as functional neurology. Subjecting a manual muscle test to various stimuli like a deep tendon stimulation or a flexor withdrawal response can help reveal any dysfunctional movement patterns. Once they have been discovered, the functional neurologist would know just what to do to get the muscles to display as they should, according to the predesigned human movement patterns.

Brain Center Integration

Two of the many different major learning centers are the cerebellum and thalamus. Both are in the brain and their jobs are similar, but they go about their ways differently. The cerebellum has been found to have between eight to twelve "on" and "off" cycles every second. The thalamus has approximately forty to fifty per second. When these two systems are in sync, they can communicate clearly. Information received

> *The primitive reflexes—e.g., the tonic neck reflex, flexor withdrawal reflex, Galant reflex, and many others—are dependent upon accurate timing mechanisms between the receptor of input and the effector of motor response. This reflex cycle generally incorporates some aspect of a muscle at either end.*

when they are both "on" is either crunched and used for motor response or filed away for future reference. The integration of data leads to optimal function.

But what happens when one or both of these two brain centers become stuck and their timing gets thrown off? What if one of the centers slows down and the other stays normal? What if both of them speed up and get out of phase with each other? Any neurological static reduces the number of times these centers are "on" at the same time, and two bits of information may never get linked. *Dys-integration*—or inappropriate integration—leads to dysfunction and pathology. That's a processing problem—a learning disability—that can be remedied by reducing or eliminating the static in the pathways.

Give this a try: Tap your fingers on a table eight to twelve individual times a second. It's hard. Now try to do it forty to fifty times in a second. That's tougher. If you can do that, then try to tap one hand eight to twelve times in a second while tapping the other hand forty to fifty times in a second. That's nearly impossible! Yet these two timing patterns must happen inside your brain every second of every minute of every day, for your entire lifetime so that our world has meaning. And that is just two of the many patterns that must constantly stay in sync with each other! The nervous system is a very busy place!

The environment can have a profound impact on timing. External influences like chemicals, allergens, sounds, and stress of many kinds can make some systems work faster and others work slower. Internal stresses can cause problems too. For optimal neurological activity and stimulation, the nerve centers should perform at their highest level. This is where functional neurology shines by finding and fixing the dysfunctional patterns and resetting the functional timing inherent to the human nervous system.

Some teachers find that there are some children in their class who just cannot sit still. They seem to be unable to stay in one place for even the shortest of periods. Besides other signs and symptoms, these kids often have trouble with pants or dresses that are too tight around their waist; they cannot stand being restricted around their middle. This phenomenon has been related to a primitive reflex called the Galant reflex.

A neuro-typical Galant reflex enables the ability to resist gravity—to stand up straight. An aberrant Galant reflex allows an abnormally flexed posture, or the inability to stand up straight. One of the main ideas of all the foregoing is that the posture must be appropriate in order for your brain to work according to its highest potential.

Alexander, a Patient*

I first met Alexander when he was eight years old. He had been previously diagnosed with learning disabilities, obsessive-compulsive disorder (OCD), and attention deficit disorder (ADD). Every one of his TNRs (see page 264) worked exactly opposite of how it was designed to work. When the muscles should have been excited they were inhibited, and when they should have been inhibited, they were excited. The same was true for every other physiological reflex I tested on him that day. It was amazing. I finally told Alexander what should happen before I retested the muscles so he would know what I expected, but it made no difference. His parents wondered how that could be. I explained that we were witnessing a neurologically mistimed cord and brain relative to gravity, and the display was directly related to the unpredictability of Alexander's final common pathway.

We used the same tool—manual muscle testing (MMT)—for every test we did. MMT is a functional neurology tool that lets us observe how the muscles respond to each known reflex test. This technique is highly effective since the brain receives its primary input from muscles and joints. The brain receives input from other areas too, but by far the highest priority stimulation to the brain comes from the muscles and joints.

After we diagnosed and treated Alexander's brain according to its unique needs, we retested his reflexes and found that they displayed themselves predictably. When his muscles were supposed to contract, they contracted. When they were supposed to relax, they relaxed.

Although the reflexes were working again, there remained a lot of work to do—specific therapy to build resistance and eliminate adaptation—but we were all encouraged as each functional test demonstrated that our techniques could get his brain working as it should relative to gravity. The point is that when the muscles work according to their original programming, we can say that the brain is receiving a clear input, and the system is static-free.

A fully functional nervous system is "neurologese" for happy.

* Alexander is not this patient's real name.

Double-Edged Learning

Recall that resistance and adaptation are the result of what the nervous system has "learned." Again, learning is the result of the input that comes to the brain and the outflow that cascades from it. Resistance is a positive outcome of a balanced input and builds endurance, while adaptation is a negative effect of progressive neurological dysfunction that always leads to a pathological response.

The consequences of neurological learning are double edged; they can either build the nervous system up or tear it down. The more appropriate incoming signals give the greatest neurological benefit. If your nervous system's function were like a television, you would probably want an HD picture. Do you remember the early days of television when each set needed rabbit ears? The sound and the picture quality could become so snowy that it was troublesome to watch for too long. Do you remember having to stand in one place holding the rabbit ears to get a clear enough picture to watch a program? It is not like that these days. Today, people watch the clear picture of HD television because it is so clear and crisp.

Proper and reciprocal nerve signals are much like having an HD picture on your neurological television. The high-density picture represents an efficient signal, while the snowy, staticky picture of a television with rabbit ears is outdated and hard to watch.

Positive neurological learning—the learning that encourages endurance—builds a stronger and healthier nervous system. An example would be when the TNRs and DTRs turn muscles on and off as they should. But negative neurological learning—the kind that sets pathways up for failure—generates static that leads to dysfunction.

Muscles learn; they have memory, and they can also forget. Among other essential components, muscles need calcium to contract, and they use energy—in the form of ATP—to relax. A working muscle should have an appropriate blood flow that supplies plenty of nutrients—i.e., calcium—and available oxygen to make energy that enables continuous contraction and relaxation.

However, when the sensory signals from the muscles and joints conflict, the brain receives input that is contrary to its originally programmed expectations and generates a motor response—based on the erroneous sensory input—that is itself erroneous, thus encouraging a hazardous loop of adaptive sensory and motor responses. That eventually leads to the muscle's forgetfulness; the muscle is unable to endure to meet its metabolic demands, so it fails. This leads to an anaerobic condition characterized by the breakdown of not only the joint's structural stability, but also the normal metabolic cycles that should otherwise support joint function—muscle fatigue, joint breakdown, "learning" issues and pain. Remember Alexander? His nervous system was so full of static that each movement reinforced a negative result.

Muscles with a strong resistance to their environment are said to be aerobic; they perform and persist in the presence of oxygen. Aerobic muscles are more likely to have the endurance to meet the demands placed on them.

Synchronized pathways are functionally durable. Coordinated nerve signals, whether they are in the cord or in the brain itself, encourage functional integrity and structural stability. Conversely, mistimed pathways—those pathways whose plasticity encourages other-than human functional display—no matter where they are, only end up in dysfunction and joint instability.

A Case in Point

> When I ask patients how they feel they often tell me, "Well, I would not be here if I felt good." People wonder why they should see a doctor if they have no pain. While pain is the number one reason people seek a doctor, serious dysfunction can often be painless. Nevertheless, dysfunction leads to pathology.

Meet Tom (not his real name), a very physically fit twenty-seven-year-old male who was working out in his usual gym. He did the same routine he had done for years, and he felt good when he finished. A friend asked him to play basketball, and off they went.

While walking onto the court dribbling a basketball, Tom's

Achilles tendon suddenly *snapped* for no apparent reason, and down he went in tremendous pain. What could have caused such a breakdown?

Walking and dribbling a basketball is not the issue. The issue is timing. Simple movement when it exceeds the capacity of the muscles and joints to work according to their original intention, eventually fails, leading to injury. Because there was too much static, the muscle was directed to contract when it should have relaxed. If natural performance comes from properly timed nerve signals in the cord, then it is reasonable to assume that Tom's Achilles trauma was from mistimed nerve signals. The accumulated stress placed an instantaneous burden on his ankle joint that exceeded its capacity and the muscle snapped!

Every muscle contraction sends input to the cord so the cord can know where the muscle is and what the muscle is doing. The cord assimilates all that input and responds with commands for the next set of

> *Tom experienced acute pain as a result of untimely nerve signals to and from his muscles, cord and brain.*

actions practically instantaneously. Some signals tell the muscles to contract and others tell them to relax, and even others control the blood flow to the working muscles. Either way, muscles respond to the commands from the cord.

> *The autonomic nervous system is responsible for the nervous system's survival.*

If the cord signals are organized according to their original design, then the muscles work reciprocally. However, if the cord is mistimed due to some input error—either from the local muscle-cord-muscle loops or those that come from the loops that go through the brain and back—the muscles get out of sync with an increased probability of joint trauma and pain.

A dysfunctional nervous system is not always accompanied by pain. Do not wait for pain! Pain

> *Blood supplies the fuel and oxygen necessary for muscles to do the work of contracting and relaxing, and it removes the waste products that are generated as a result of that work.*

is not always the end result! Nerve signals can silently misfire, but pain-free function does not mean error-free performance.

An accumulation of timing errors eventually leads to the experience of pain with seemingly normal movement. Functional cues can lead the functional neurologist right to the problem and, in many cases, fix it with non-invasive techniques well before it starts to hurt.

Learning, Unrelated to Books or Classes

When we use the term, "learning," we are not necessarily meaning the increased knowledge that comes from books. The learning we are talking about here is more from experiences. The learning we refer to has to do with the subconscious or reflexive response to nerve activity.

A few of the cord's autonomic functions are to provide blood to the muscles and skin upon demand, and regulate functional body temperature through the sweat glands and hair. The cord reflexes are controlled from the top down, by the brain's outflow.

Did you know that research has proved that a person's ability to learn is directly related to their ability to move about on two feet, and vice versa? It all comes down to 1) the ability to harness the effects of gravity, 2) the timing of the brain centers that move us from place to place, and 3) the ability of the nervous system to adapt to an upright posture.

Certain parts of the human brain set us apart from animals. Besides other obvious differences, humans walk on two legs, and the animals walk on all fours. The more we humans can energize the centers that keep us upright, the better we can perform, and that leads to a greater ability to express our individual learning potentials.

The benefits of exercise are much more important for the brain than they are for the muscles.

Autonomic Involvement

Muscles can only do useful work when supported by a highly organized spinal cord and brain. When reflexes work with an efficient reciprocity—that preprogrammed give-and-take pattern associated with the contraction of one muscle and the simultaneous relaxation of the muscle that opposes it—their display is functional, or effortless. But when the muscles that surround a particular joint try to contract or relax simultaneously—i.e., the co-contraction of competing muscles, or when muscles lose their reciprocal design—stability wanes, setting up the muscles for movement errors, the structure for functional breakdown, and the whole body for systemic disorder.

These dysfunctional patterns are often fixable. If we continue with the tonic neck reflex idea, we can test each muscle's ability to contract in order to understand if its dynamics are reciprocal. If the muscles respond functionally—i.e., if the muscles contract and relax as anticipated—then we can say that the nervous system (the cord and brain) is able to update the information fast enough to maintain integrity. But if the muscles respond in any way other than as we would anticipate, then we could say that the nerve signals to and from the cord are unable to update themselves fast enough. This represents a loss of cord integrity, and the muscles turn *off*. The point is that even dysfunctional pathways have plasticity; if plasticity exists, it persists.

> *Of all the nerve signals that leave the brain and go to the body, only 10% go to the muscles. Up to 90% of the brain's outflow goes to autonomic controls.*

A Review of Cord Activity

Recall the twelve events that happen when a nerve signal enters the cord. Remember that the most important event is to provide fuel and oxygen to the tissues in order to support life. The autonomic—or "automatic"—nervous system is responsible for the means of survival.

In general, the autonomic system is responsible for maintaining blood pressure, heart rate, body temperature, digestion, breathing, sleep and wakefulness, glandular function, and several other processes necessary for life. A key to youth and longevity is to maintain functional autonomics. Without autonomic controls, life would gradually diminish and eventually cease altogether.

What Went Wrong?

> *Most chiropractors are trained to adjust the spine by hand, but sometimes that is the least important treatment to give. The brain uses the spine for adaptive measures and taking away that adaptation may lead to more complicated means of handling a problem.*

Structural failure begins when a muscle's demands exceed its capacity. When we overwork or overuse a muscle, or force a muscle to perform beyond its ability to keep up with the endurance demands placed on it, muscle fatigue sets in, stability suffers and this jeopardizes autonomic performance. That familiar burn of muscle work is the nervous system's way of telling you to stop. When a muscle "burns," it is physiologically saying that it needs more blood and oxygen; it has reached the limits of its aerobic capacity and it is about to quit. Fatigue, jerky or irregular muscle contractions indicate that the functional limits of the muscle have been reached, and continuing past this point contributes to a functional joint breakdown that eventually results in pathology. While that burn can be useful at the right time, it leads to pathology in the absence of an established aerobic foundation.

Since structural failure represents a compromise of normal nerve signal controls, this also leads to an erosion of autonomic controls; we call this *autonomic escape*. When the autonomic nervous system allows some display that should have otherwise been controlled, we observe signs and symptoms that represent pathology. An example should be the red lines that form on the skin after scratching an itch. This redness is an engorgement of the capillaries near the surface of the skin, and should not red-

> *The autonomic nervous system affects heart rate, digestion, respiratory rate, salivation, perspiration, pupillary dilation, micturition (urination), and sexual arousal. Whereas most of its actions are involuntary, some, such as breathing, work in tandem with the conscious mind.*

den so quickly. Some redness may be normal, but an acute, bright redness is an escape of autonomic controls that should keep the engorgement from happening. Resetting the nerve signal controls with functional neurological techniques can often reset the autonomic response and reestablish the normal vascular display.

When a muscle is pushed beyond its ability to do useful work, fatigue sets in and stability suffers, and instability and fatigue both jeopardize autonomic performance. This is the much too common result of exercise that goes beyond the muscle's capacity, i.e., shakiness, nausea, tachycardia, etc.

Battered nerve signals are not necessarily painful, but their results eventually lead to neurological breakdown. Fatigued muscles still send signals to the cord, but instead of supporting the preprogrammed human movement patterns, they create and encourage plasticity consistent with dysfunction, resulting in erroneous cord effects.

Functional Autonomics

Adding anaerobic exercise on top of an unstable or non-existent aerobic base can be injurious to both the muscles and brain.

One might consider that the human brain controls the muscles, but that is only partly true. Of all the neurological signals that leave the brain, only 10% of those signals go to muscle. Ninety percent of the brain's outflow is meant to influence the autonomic nervous system, which controls *all* body processes. To gauge the effectiveness of the nervous system, it is essential to monitor the functional autonomics.

Human Performance

In one human performance class, we calculated the patient's target aerobic heart rate (according to Maffetone), and then tested their muscles with manual muscle testing techniques to measure their degree of functional stability. The patient was then asked to run around the room to quickly bring their heart rate into their target zone, and then get back on the table to be retested. The muscle tests showed that the previously weak muscles were still weak, and amazingly so were the previously strong muscles.

After the patient's heart rate returned to rest, we retested the muscles again and noted any differences from the previous tests. The patient was again asked to bring their heart rate into its aerobic target zone, but to gradually increase their heart rate over a ten- to fifteen-minute period by walking at an increasing pace. This time when the patient got back on the table, the previously weak muscles were strong and the previously strong muscles stayed strong.

> *In one patient who had an aerobic deficiency, the strong muscles became weak and the weak muscles stayed weak. But when they addressed their exercise correctly, their weak muscles became strong and the strong muscles stayed strong indicating that the nervous system had greater efficiency, and so did the brain.*

> *Centerline structures influence the centerline brain, and vice versa. The most centerline human structure is the spine (and the cord that runs through it).*

The inference of the first test was that the muscles weakened because their cord and brain-based autonomic stamina was unable to meet the functional demands placed on them; blood and oxygen could not be shunted to them relative to their need. Conversely, the second test indicated that the autonomic system properly met the demand of the muscles because the blood and oxygen were able to reach the muscles according to their demand.

The surrounding influences from the cord provided the stimulation for the autonomic support, but the more significant influence on the ventral horn actually came down from the brain. Recall that every nerve signal that reaches the cord generates twelve cord-related events at the same cord level where the signal arrived, but each of these events in each of the cord segments is regulated from the highest priority controls that come from the brain.

The muscles give input to the cord and brain, and the brain and cord tell the muscles what to do. When the muscles, cord, and brain are all on the same page insofar as the autonomic controls are concerned, order gives rise to order and stability is the rule. However, if just one of these three components gets out of sync, dysfunction is the ultimate result. This leads to disorder, pain, and eventual degeneration.

Reset Your Brain's Timing

> *The brain is the nexus of all body processes, and the benefits of exercise are much more important for the brain than they are for the muscles.*

The primary brain input comes from the nerves that are within the muscles, and the nerves that surround the joints—both called proprioceptors. It takes some sort of neurological input via structural change to affect the deep nociception-control centers of the brain in a positive and beneficial way. The point being: do not rely solely on pain killers, muscle relaxers, or vitamins to take away your pain when the problem is the result of brain-timing errors.

A basic neurological truth is that centerline structures influence the centerline brain, and vice versa. The body works as a whole unit; the

> *Remember that resistance builds functional capacity and adaptation leads to pathology.*

parts are inseparable. The human system is designed with function and survival as its main concern. So it makes sense that parts related to each other should work together and said to be homologous. For example, the eyes, tongue, and certain parts of the brain and cerebellum together with the whole spine are all hard-wired as an homologous column with the goal to resist gravity. They all have to do with balance and stability in an upright environment.

There is no more centerline human *structure* than the spine. So, to generate the best brain function it follows to make sure that your spine is working as well as it can; that all its parts are moving through their full range of motion without becoming stuck within any part of that motion. So, for better brain function, let's keep your spine and the spinal cord working, primed, and ready.

The Spinal Adjustment

> *If adapted tissues have any chance of resolving, then the essential components for their repair must be made available in a timely fashion and in the right amounts. Even then, resolution is not guaranteed.*

To most chiropractors, that means adjusting the spine. However, a functional neurologist realizes spinal dynamics more clearly. Spinal joints tend to get stuck in order to help the brain deal with a functional issue. Since the outgoing motor signals from the brain have direct influence over the muscles that move the spine, any sensory timing errors will be displayed in the motor response to the spinal joints as a subluxation—a misalignment of the vertebrae caused by muscle spasm. Taking away any subluxation has a very real possibility of removing an adaptation created by the brain in response to a particular sensory problem.

Someone might ask, "Since we have already discussed that adaptation is a progression into pathology, why would it be inappropriate to remove spinal adaptation with a chiropractic adjustment?" A very astute question. Remember, adaptation is always pathological.

According to Beardall, the stages of the adaptative cascade are progressive. Adaptation evolves when the essential components for repair are persistently unavailable. If the breakdown has not crossed the academic barrier of questionable return (somewhere between the exhaustive stage six and the degenerative stage seven), then the resolution of the adaptation has the potential to reverse itself along an equally logical path. However, if that reversal has any chance of happening, the essential components for repair must be made available in a timely manner to bring about the potential for healing, but the tissues will probably never return to their original and healthy state. A spinal adjustment, while stimulating the incoming and outgoing signals to and from the brain, can do nothing to directly address the issue of the essential components for repair. That must be done with nutrition, treatment, and specific rehabilitation.

Functional neurological treatments are designed to treat the brain, but the key is that those treatments have to be done properly in order to be effective. When it comes to movement disorders, drugs and medications have nothing to offer people with these issues. Often, drugs are used in ways other than their original intent—termed, "off-label"—in order to obtain certain responses, but no matter how it is intended every drug has side effects that can cause other problems. These problems even have their own name: tardive dyskinesia, a

The use of certain antipsychotic drugs has led to tardive dyskinesia—a number of harmful and undesired effects linked to movement disorders with a slow and belated onset. There is a potential for permanent chemical dependence leading to psychosis much worse than before treatment began, if the drug dosage is ever lowered or stopped.

Temporary withdrawal symptoms including insomnia, agitation, psychosis, and motor disorders may occur and can be mistaken for a return of the underlying condition.

difficult-to-treat disorder resulting in involuntary, repetitive body movements that have a slow or belated onset. It frequently appears after long-term or high-dose use of many very common antipsychotic drugs. It also appears in children and infants as a side effect from usage of drugs for the prevention of gastrointestinal disorders.

Treating one aspect of neurological performance with a prescription drug may lead to unintended consequences and long term disabilities in the future. Neuroleptics or antipsychotic drugs, like Abilify®, Haldol®, Risperdal®, Seroquel®, Zyprexa®, and many others; or non-neuroleptic drugs, like Elavil®, Lithium®, Prozac®, Reglan®, Zoloft®; and the recreational use of cocaine are all related to the potential onset of tardive dyskinesia.

Chiropractor versus Functional Neurologist

There is a huge difference between a regular chiropractor and a functional neurologist. When it comes to their training and therapeutic techniques, functional neurologists are highly trained to understand the makeup and inner workings of the brain and its relationship to the entire body.

> *If your brain could speak, it might say: "Please do not take matters into your own hands, or put your neurological care in the hands of someone untrained or unqualified to read and understand your big picture." Your neurological health deserves and requires a trained professional who is "neuro-lingual"—trained to read the signs, translate the signals, understand their meaning, and plan for a successful and complete neurological rehabilitation.*

Functional Neurology began within the chiropractic community as an alternative holistic specialty that deals with the functional instability of the brain and the entire nervous system, but is quickly attracting those with more traditional medical training. Functional neurologists receive specialized training in the application of neurological sciences. These specialists are skilled at stimulating a person's sensory system and monitoring the changes in the neurological response. They treat the patient according to the anticipated response; if the systems are working right, they will respond with an anticipated reaction. If not, then the treatment changes and the new response is observed. These diagnostic procedures are designed to detect and treat functional neurological changes before their adaptive progression to irreversible pathology. The goal is to restore optimal function for health and wellness, to improve autonomic balance, return hormone stability, encourage immune display, and reduce the experience of pain.

Out of the Dark Ages

Some people have another person walk on their back, others lie on some sort of roller device, and still others roll around on the floor lifting one leg or the other, hoping something in their back will pop. Most often, this is not an effective treatment. Although their back may pop, it may be that their bones are moving the wrong way, and this could potentially cause further problems—like arthritis and degenerative discs—creating more static down the road.

Massage, physical therapy, and/or exercise miss the mark when it comes to deep brain stimulation. None of these can reach the brain centers that are stimulated by coupled chiropractic adjustments to the deep bony structures because these adjustments are delivered to the deep centerline spinal structures. All other less specific therapies are stimulating only the skin and the underlying muscles.

> *Coupled movement relates to both spinal motion and a type of specific adjustive technique. Either way, coupled action indicates the spine is moving according to its original design.*

When determined to be appropriate for the condition, the most appropriate therapeutic signal to the brain comes as a result of coupled chiropractic adjustments, which are different from other spinal adjustments that quickly twist the patient's spine. Coupled adjustments are quite powerful and are done without a twist. Twisting the neck has the potential to cause joint related problems over a long period, and that can lead to brain-related issues—since centerline structures are all related.

Coupled chiropractic adjustments are the specialty of functional neurologists. We understand when and how to, and the benefits of adjusting the spine according to its purposeful and preprogrammed movement patterns, and that adjustment's effects on the spinal cord, brain, and ultimately the muscles. Uncoupled adjustments, on the other hand, have a very high probability of producing both structural and functional breakdown.

The Consequences of Untreated Static

> *People who habitually adjust their own back or neck may get relief from discomfort but that may be because the joints are moving the wrong way, which dulls their ability to perceive how they feel, so they think they feel better when in fact their nervous system is further compromised.*

When imbalanced movement persists, your nervous system disconnects from how it should work and falters to a "new normal" that accumulates neurological static and the dysplasticity that goes with it. The preprogrammed patterns of human movement are overcome by these staticky signals, which functionally take over. What should have been kept from happening now becomes a "new" display. Although this new reality may very well be pain-free, it is nonetheless pathological because it is other than what would be considered to be a normal pattern—muscles now contract when they should be relaxed, and relax when they should contract. Yet over time, these new patterns are tolerated as "normal." With time, the functionally abnormal human nervous system adapts into degeneration and beyond, leaving a compromised structure and function in its wake. The structural breakdown leads to the decline of brain powers with eventual emotional demise. The longer this disconnect persists the longer and more difficult it is to rehabilitate, if it can be saved at all.

Summary

Do you find yourself struggling against gravity? Are you often caught by gravity? If gravity is your nemesis rather than your ally, call a functional neurologist right away. *Functional neurologists speak fluent "neurologese!"*

Functional reciprocity is the key to human fitness in both body and brain. Vigorous health is built on equal and opposite reactions of body systems. A push should always be met with a pull; balance is always linked with

> *If your brain is having trouble breathing, if it is toxic, if it stumbles over its words, and if there is too much static, then your nervous system is functioning in a way that is "other-than-human."*

counterbalance. The body's reaction to its environment is always dynamic and the brain's experience is always plastic. When the body and brain respond to its environment properly, that response is always according to preprogrammed human response patterns. Relatable movements are always coordinated and reciprocal, being made possible by an intact nervous system composed of synergistic primitive reflex patterns that produce the more mature human nervous fabric.

Nerve static is at the crux of breakdown and disease. This static generally displays itself as a malfunction of appropriate movement. Movement error creates abnormal sensory input that is perceived as conflict when the nervous system's preprogramming anticipates a more appropriate signal. Any signal other than that which is preprogrammed should always be considered to be pathological, and it is perceived by the nervous system as static.

How is the fabric of your nervous system doing? How much static is there within your preprogramming and what is its effect? Nerve static is never good and always has negative consequences. Neurological noisiness gradually tears at the fabric of our nervous system, making us more prone to physical injury, sickness, disease, and pain. Without reciprocity the human nervous system adapts to its dysfunctional condition and eventually disintegrates.

Let's be sure your brain and functional reflex patterns are static-free and working according to their original design. There are simple and painless ways to examine you for any movement errors that

> *The primitive reflexes are generally those that appear at some point during gestation or after birth, and eventually become incorporated into the maturing nervous system.*

might keep you from resisting gravity properly and being as healthy as your original design.

SOME FINAL THOUGHTS

If Your Brain Could Speak, It Might Say...

Well, there you have it. We have discovered that if your brain could speak, it would probably have plenty to say. Would it speak well of you or would it complain? Might your nervous system say that it was having trouble breathing? Detoxifying? Conversing? Working? It is quite probable that your nervous system is trying to tell you, "Hey, let's do things differently!"

DO NOT EAT:
• Hydrogenated oils
• Trans-fatty acids
• Artificial coloring
• Artificial flavoring
• Too much sugar
• Junk foods

It is fitting for each of us to find a doctor who is able to interpret our brain's needs clearly and teach us how to supply the essential components of these needs right away. To get the help you might need, seek out a licensed functional neurologist or some other alternative healthcare professional who can help you read your body's signs. Participate with that doctor and learn how to speak fluent "Neurologese."

We have learned several concepts about what your brain might say if it could speak. Now it is time to apply these things that will make a difference in the way you feel and the way you act.

Learn to breathe. Change your diet. Cleanse your system. Drink clean water. Sleep. Go out and exercise according to your individual needs to be sure your muscles are sending the right kind of signals to your brain. These actions will provide obvious benefits. In the place of saying, "I can't breathe," you brain will say, "Ahh, fresh air!" Instead of, "I can't take it anymore," your brain will say, "Now I can handle it!" Rather than saying,

"I lost the words," your brain will say, "Thanks for listening!" And rather than it saying, "Stop the static," your brain will say, "Now, that's clearer!"

I know that when it is all said and done, your brain will say, "thank you for taking such good care of me."

Functional neurology can help you. Until your next appointment, I hope you stay well, now and always!

EAT RIGHT

Eat organic, fresh, unprocessed foods as often as possible.

Some healthy foods:

- *Organic dairy and meat*
- *Wild salmon*
- *All fresh fruits and vegetables*
- *Brown rice*
- *Rolled oats*
- *Barley*
- *Millet*
- *Nuts (pecans, almonds, macadamia, hazel, Brazil, etc.)*
- *Seeds (walnuts, sunflower, pumpkin, sesame, etc.)*
- *Berries*
- *Beans (pinto, black, navy, red, fava, kidney, etc.)*
- *Flaxseed oil*

GLOSSARY

Acetylcholine: Abbreviated ACh, is a neurotransmitter in both the peripheral nervous system (PNS) and central nervous system (CNS) in humans.

Adaptogen: A metabolic regulator with a normalizing effect; it increases the ability of an organism to adapt to environmental factors, and to avoid damage from such factors.

Adipose: Body fat; loose connective tissue composed of roughly only 80% fat. Adipose tissue stores energy in the form of lipids, although it also cushions and insulates the body.

Aldosterone: A steroid hormone produced by the adrenal gland. It increases reabsorption of ions and water in the kidney—increasing blood volume and, therefore, increasing blood pressure.

Allopathy: Also known as allopathic medicine; a term regularly used by proponents of alternative medicine and alternative medical practices to differentiate their philosophy from that of the broad caregory of medicine generally referred to as western medicine and its mainstream medical use of pharmacologically active substances to treat or suppress symptoms or pathophysiologic processes of diseases or conditions.

ANP: see Arterial natriuretic peptide

Anthocyanidins: Powerful, specific bioflavonoid compounds responsible for the pigmentation of various fruits and vegetables; they are widely known for their antioxidant properties.

Antigravity muscle: Those muscles that are able to resist and endure the effects of gravity; they tend to be aerobic; extensor muscles.

Anti-neoplastic: The ability to inhibit or prevent development of a neoplasm; checking maturation and proliferation of malignant cells.

Asteraceae: Several plants of the daisy-like family including arnica, artemisia, feverfew, tansy, and yarrow.

Atrial natriuretic peptide: A powerful vasodilator, and a protein hormone secreted by heart muscle cells.

Autonomic nervous system: That part of the human nervous system that functions without you having to do anything; monitors and manages such processes as heart rate, blood pressure, body temperature, sleep and wakefulness, fluid balance, and more.

Axon: Also known as a nerve fiber; a long, slender projection of a nerve cell, or neuron, that typically conducts electrical signals away from the neuron's cell body.

Basal ganglia: A group of nuclei found below the cerebral cortex that act as an organized functional unit. They are strongly connected with the cerebral cortex, thalamus and other brain areas and associated with a variety of functions, including voluntary motor control, procedural learning relating to routine behaviors or "habits," eye movements, and cognitive, emotional functions.

Bioavailable: The measure of how easily a drug or other substance is absorbed or becomes available at the site of biological activity after it is consumed by a person.

Bioavailability: The act of being bioavailable.

Cardiomyopathy: Also known as "heart muscle disease"; the measurable deterioration of heart muscle function for any reason.

Carcinogenic: The ability of any substance to disrupt the normal cellular metabolic processes and produce cancerous cells.

Carnosic acid: A natural compound found in rosemary and common sage.

Catecholamines:	Hormones produced by the adrenal glands that are released into the blood during times of physical or emotional stress. The major catecholamines are dopamine, norepinephrine, and epinephrine (which used to be called adrenalin).
Chiropractic:	That complementary and alternative branch of the art and science of healthcare that is concerned with the diagnosis, treatment and prevention of disorders of the neuromusculoskeletal system and the effects of these disorders on general health; it is based on the belief that the nervous system is the primary avenue of physiological influence for the treatment of disease conditions; the main treatment techniques involve manual therapy, including manipulation of the spine, other joints, and soft tissues; treatment also includes exercises and health and lifestyle counseling; traditional chiropractic assumes that a vertebral subluxation interferes with the body's innate intelligence.
Cobalamin:	One aspect of the Vitamin B complex; an especially important vitamin for maintaining healthy nerve cells, and it helps in the production of DNA and RNA, the body's genetic material.
Cofactors:	A biological substance that works with an enzyme to increase the rate of a (bio)chemical reaction.
Cortisol:	A steroid hormone produced by the adrenal gland in response to stress and a low level of blood glucocorticoids. Its primary functions are to increase blood sugar; suppress the immune system; aids in fat, protein and carbohydrate metabolism.
Coupled movement:	A chiropractic term relating to between three and several spinal motor units moving harmoniously in different planes and on different axes.
Covalent:	A chemical bond that is characterized by the stable balance of attractive and repulsive forces.

Cytocrome P450: The cytochrome p450 enzymes are a powerful detoxification system; our first line of detoxification that flushes poisons that arise from the diet, breath, drug consumption, poisonous compounds in plants, carcinogens formed during cooking, and environmental pollutants.

Deafferentation: A reduction of sensory input to the cord and/or brain.

Dendrite: The branched projections of a neuron that can conduct the electrochemical stimulation from another nerve cell to the rest of the neuron.

Desaturated: Also referred to as long-chain polyunsaturated fatty acids; omega-3, omega-6, and omega-9 fatty acids.

Endocrinologist: A medical specialist who has advanced fields of study in the disorders of glands and hormones, and their related disorders.

Endorphins: Special neurotransmitters that transmit electrical signals within the nervous system; stress and pain are the two most common factors leading to the release of endorphins; at least twenty types of endorphins have been demonstrated in the human pituitary gland, in other parts of the brain, or distributed throughout the nervous system.

Fast twitch fibers: Those muscles that are characterized by the inability to use oxygen; they are anaerobic, white, type I, fast twitch muscles; they have few mitochondria and are unable to endure the effects of gravity.

Final common pathway: Found in the anterior horn of the spinal cord; the very last possible location that all sensory and motor pathways can come together to influence an alpha-motoneuron to the periphery. The "final common pathway" for central nervous system control of behavior.

Fixation:	The immobilization of three spinal motor units as one, making them work together instead of allowing the normal freedom seen with coupled motion; a fixation can lead to significant spinal degenerative changes compared to the mobile joints.
Furan:	A colorless solvent or resin used in some segments of the chemical manufacturing; a toxic chemical that is found in very small amounts in the environment, including air, water soil and some foods; thought to produce a wide range of carcinogenic and mutagenic effects in laboratory animals and humans.
Glial cell:	Commonly referred to as the nervous system's glue; non-neuronal cells that maintain homeostasis, form myelin, and provide support and protection for neurons in the brain, and for neurons in other parts of the nervous system such as in the autonomic nervous system.
Goitrogens:	Substances that have the ability to produce an enlarged thyroid gland—a goiter; able to suppress the function of the thyroid gland by interfering with iodine uptake.
Hemisphericity:	Differences in firing rates between the left and right sides of the brain.
Homeostasis:	Maintenance of relatively stable internal physiological conditions, i.e., temperature or pH of blood—in higher animals under fluctuating environmental conditions.
Hypolipemic:	The condition relating to a low concentration of lipids or fats in the blood.
Inflammation:	An essential body defense necessary for immune response.
In vitro:	Literally means "within glass"; living components having been isolated from their usual biological context; colloquially, commonly referred to as "test tube experiments."
In vivo:	Refers to work that is conducted with living organisms in their normal, intact state.

Ionizing radiation:	Ionizing radiation is energy composed of particles that individually carry enough energy to cause the release of an electron from an atom or a molecule, ionizing it; acquiring an electric charge or changing an existing charge. Ionizing radiation is generated through nuclear reactions, either artificial or natural, by very high temperature.
Isomer:	One of many different classes of compounds with the same molecular formula but different structural formulas; they do not necessarily share similar properties.
Limiting amino acids:	The essential amino acid found in the smallest quantity in the foodstuff.
Mutagenic:	An agent that can induce or increase the frequency of changes in an organism's genetic sequence; a chemical, ultraviolet light, or a radioactive element.
Myelination:	A special insulating layer of material that forms a sheath around only the axon of a neuron. It is essential for the proper functioning of the nervous system.
Naturopathy:	Also referred to as Naturopathic Medicine; that alternative medical branch of the art and science of healthcare that is based on the use of any and all natural methods that positively influence the vital aspects of human physiology including such avenues as metabolism, reproduction, growth, and adaptation in the treatment of disease; it favors a holistic approach with non-invasive treatment by encouraging minimal use of surgery and drugs.
Neoplasm:	A mass of tissue that grows in a (new) way other than that of normal tissue.
Neuron:	An electrically excitable cell that processes and transmits information by electrical and chemical signaling.
Neuroplasticity:	Rewire and rework the brain; creates new circuitry and making it stronger to take over; no morphological changes; regenerative.

Nociception:	The unconscious recognition of mechanical, chemical or thermal changes that have the potential to create the perception of pain; these signals travel at about a half meter (or approximately 18 inches) per second.
Osteopathy:	That branch of the art and science of healthcare that emphasizes the connectivity of the blood vascular system as the primary avenue to influence human physiology for the treatment of disease conditions; it recognizes the body's ability to heal itself; it is the role of the osteopath to facilitate that process, principally by the practice of manual and manipulative therapy.
PDCAAS:	The "Protein Digestibility Corrected Amino Acid Score"; the method by which the World Health Organization evaluates protein value. It's a newer model, and it's based on the amino acid requirements of humans, specifically children.
Peptides:	Short chains of repeating amino acids linked by bonds that are not particularly strong.
Peroxidase:	A large family of enzymes that typically cause or accelerate a reaction.
Phase One Detoxification:	The first of two phases of liver detoxification that uses oxygen (oxidation) and enzymes to burn toxins; a breakdown process that separates components of larger molecules and makes them water soluble to be more easily excreted from the body by the kidneys or the liver.
Phase Two Detoxification:	The second of two phases of liver detoxification; eliminates breakdown products from phase one, called conjugation; oxidized chemicals are combined with sulfur, specific amino acids, or organic acids, and then excreted in bile; negatively affected by nutritional deficiency, toxic exposures, medications such as acetaminophen (brand name Tylenol®), alcohol consumption, and low protein intake that deplete glutathione which is needed for acetaminophen detoxification.

Phytochemicals:	Any one of an estimated 10,000 natural plant biochemical compounds; responsible for color; generally refers to those chemicals that may have biological significance but are not established as essential nutrients; having the potential to affect diseases such as cancer, stroke or metabolic syndrome; potential health benefits of phytochemicals may best come from consumption of whole foods.
Phytonutrients:	(Synonymous with phytochemicals.)
Plasticity:	Your brain responds to experience and training either in appropriate or inappropriate ways.
Prefrontal cortex (PFC):	The front-most part of the frontal lobes of the brain, lying in front of the motor and premotor areas; implicated in executive function [differentiate among conflicting thoughts, determine good and bad, better and best, same and different, future consequences of current activities, working toward a defined goal, prediction of outcomes, expectation based on actions, and social "control" (the ability to suppress urges that, if not suppressed, could lead to socially unacceptable outcomes)], planning complex cognitive behavior, personality expression, decision making, and moderating social behavior; the basic activity is considered to be orchestration of thoughts and actions in accordance with internal goals.
Proprioception:	"One's own," "individual" and perception; the unconscious recognition of a joint's position in space and the strength of effort to move that joint; the automatic realizing the position of a body part; these signals travel at about 120 meter (or approximately one and one third football fields) per second.
Proprioceptors:	Those receptors that perceive proprioception.
Protein Digestibility-Corrected Amino Acid Score:	(see PDCAAS)

Protein-Energy Malnutrition:	Any one of several metabolic disorders where the cellular imbalance between the supply of nutrients and energy, and the body's demand for them to ensure growth, maintenance, and specific functions becomes compromised, leading to disease [The World Health Organization (WHO)].
Reciprocal(ly):	Inversely related or proportional; opposite; something that is equivalent, a counterpart, or complement to something else.
Reflex:	An involuntary, almost instantaneous movement in response to a stimulus; generally attributed to the peripheral nervous system when decreased and to the central nervous system when lively or exaggerated.
Slow twitch muscles:	Those muscles that are characterized by the use of oxygen; they are aerobic, red, type II, slow twitch muscles; they have copious mitochondria and are able to endure the effects of gravity; antigravity muscles.
Spinal joints:	(See spinal motor unit)
Spinal motor unit:	Two adjacent vertebra, an intervertebral disc and their intervening joints are called a spinal motor unit; all the spinal motor units must work in a coupled fashion in order for the spine to move.
Spontaneous discharge:	The unplanned firing of a nerve impulse that results when the nerve cell's resting membrane potential reaches the threshold of discharge.
Subluxation:	The term for a joint whose range of motion is limited within its normal range, yet is unable to move through its normal range; an incomplete or partial dislocation. It is not always visible on an x-ray or other type of radiograph.
Superoxide dismutase (SOD):	An enzyme that breaks a specific and unstable oxygen molecule into its component parts; an important antioxidant defense in nearly all cells exposed to oxygen.
Surface ectoderm:	The outermost of the three primary germ layers of an embryo, from which the epidermis, nervous tissue, and, in vertebrates, sense organs develop.

Symptoms: A body's expression of its wisdom and should be understood, not suppressed.

Synthetic vitamins: Any one or a combination of distilled or fractionated vitamin components recognized by authoritarian agencies as having a role in human nutrition.

Tardive dyskinesia: A form of aberrant movement with a slow or belated onset; a disorder resulting in involuntary, repetitive body movements; frequently appears after long-term or high-dose use of antipsychotic drugs, or in children and infants as a side effect from usage of drugs for gastrointestinal disorders.

Tissue(s): A cooperative group of cells that may have varying identity, but arise from the same fundamental origin designed to carry out a specific function; a level of cellular organization between cells and a complete organism. Organs are formed by the functional grouping together of multiple tissues.

Uncoupled movement: Relating to an inharmonious or aberrant movement pattern between three and several spinal motor units; sprained and/or strained movement through different planes and on different axes.

Venous insufficiency: A medical condition where the veins cannot pump enough oxygen-poor blood back to the heart from the lower extremities because of damaged or "incompetent" valves in the legs.

Xenobiotics: Any foreign organic compounds not produced in metabolism; a chemical compound (as a drug, pesticide, or carcinogen) that is foreign to a living organism.

INDEX

311

M

Y

Z

CPSIA information can be obtained at www.ICGtesting.com
Printed in the USA
BVOW081535200613

323821BV00001B/2/P